Back Sense

Back Sense

A Revolutionary Approach to Halting the Cycle of Chronic Back Pain

Ronald D. Siegel, Psy.D.,
Michael H. Urdang,
and Douglas R. Johnson, M.D.

Broadway Books
New York

BROADWAY

Broadway Books titles may be purchased for business or promotional use or for special sales. For information, please write to: Special Markets Department, Random House, Inc., 1540 Broadway, New York, NY 10036.

Visit our Web site at www.broadwaybooks.com

Library of Congress Cataloging-in-Publication Data
Siegel, Ronald D.
Back sense : a revolutionary approach to halting the cycle of chronic back pain / Ronald D. Siegel, Michael H. Urdang, and Douglas R. Johnson.
p. ; cm.
Includes bibliographical references and index.
1. Backache. 2. Backache—Psychological aspects. 3. Backache—Treatment. I. Title: Revolutionary approach to halting the cycle of chronic back pain. II. Urdang, Michael H. III. Johnson, Douglas R. IV. Title.
[DNLM: 1. Back Pain—therapy. 2. Chronic Disease. 3. Mental Healing. WE 720 S571b 2000]
RD771.B217 S55 2000
617.5'64—dc21

00-045466

FIRST EDITION

DESIGNED BY DEBORAH KERNER/DANCING BEARS DESIGN

ISBN 0-7679-0636-5
01 02 03 04 05 10 9 8 7 6 5 4 3 2 1

For our families,

and our patients

CONTENTS

ACKNOWLEDGMENTS

Many people have made substantial contributions to the creation of this book.

We would, first of all, like to thank the researchers and clinicians whose work laid the foundation for the Back Sense program. In particular, we'd like to acknowledge Dr. John Sarno, a pioneer in understanding the role of the mind in back pain; and Dr. James Rainville, who has developed practical, proven programs of functional restoration and introduced us to the crucial importance of resuming full physical activity in curing back pain. We would also like to thank Dr. Eugenio Martinez, who has worked with us in perfecting an integrated approach to treatment, and to thank as well the numerous other colleagues who have shared their ideas and encouraged us in our work.

We are very grateful to the many people at the Doubleday Broadway Publishing Group who have helped bring the book to completion, especially to our editor, Patricia Medved, who suggested innumerable improvements to the manuscript; to Gerald Howard, who was the first to see the completed manuscript and eased our first-time-author anxieties; and to Jennifer Griffin, who originally brought us to Broadway Books.

Our agent, Ira Silverberg, and his colleagues at Donadio & Olson, have offered us great assistance and encouragement in seeing the work through from initial inspiration to completed book.

For their astute counsel and aid during several stages of the book's evolution, we'd like to thank Jennifer Brehl, Mark Dalton, Alan Litner, and Deborah Weisgall.

For their help in reading and refining the manuscript, we would like to thank Dr. Parakrama Ananta, Fred Armstrong, Florie Arons, Dr. Michele Bograd, Shari Duane, Joyce Jansen, Robert Jenne, David Johnson, Dr. Eugenio Martinez, Ellen Matathia, Dr. Andrew Mazur, Dr. James Rainville, Joan Stoddard, and others who prefer to remain anonymous.

We are also especially indebted to our patients, who have taught us so much about the treatment of back pain and have actively helped us to develop this program.

Finally, we cannot say enough to adequately thank our families for their considerable patience, sound advice, and enduring support: Mary Ann Dalton; Christa, Anna, Michael, and Sarah Johnson; Gina Arons; and Alexandra and Julia Siegel.

PART 1

UNDERSTANDING CHRONIC BACK PAIN

CHAPTER 1

A NEW APPROACH TO BACK PAIN

BACK PAIN BULLETIN!

If you've been suffering with back pain, we don't need to tell you just how bad it can get. It's an ordeal. You suffer, your family suffers, your friends suffer, your work suffers. Your whole quality of life can take a nosedive. There are millions of other people with the same problem, but that doesn't make it any easier to handle. We know that it's hard to believe, but the book you hold in your hands can help—and help a lot. It's about an exciting new approach to understanding and treating chronic back pain that integrates the very best from both "traditional" and "alternative" medicine so you can resume your normal life as soon as possible. It is based on an explosion of recent scientific research that leads to a whole new way of understanding and treating back pain that has become a chronic problem (lingered more than a couple of months).

Simply put, the book makes three major points:

1. The cause of most chronic back pain is generally misunderstood by both sufferers and the medical community. It is usually thought to be the result of damaged or defective parts in the back. This is a perfectly natural assumption, but, strange as this seems, it simply isn't true. A great deal of scientific research has been done on chronic back pain, and the findings point in a completely different direction. So what does cause chronic back pain? The evidence tells us that while the problem may start with a physical injury or strain, those things usually heal quickly on their own. Tight muscles cause the pain to last, and stress is to blame for tight muscles—stress over pain, worries about the future, disappointments over unsuccessful cures, fears of surgery, anxieties about medical bills, problems at work, unhappiness over strained relationships. *The pain is certainly not "all in your head." We know that it is completely real.* Muscle tension and spasms can cause intense pain.

2. Most current back pain treatment methods don't work very well because they misunderstand the real cause of the pain. Again the research contradicts typical medical practice. If you are like most people, you've taken your back troubles to one or more doctors. You may have been told to rest, take medicine, or attend "back school." Perhaps you've tried special cushions, braces, physical therapy, a chiropractor, or even surgery. You're probably very careful to avoid reinjuring yourself. Some of these measures may have helped to a degree, but they probably haven't solved your problem entirely or you wouldn't be reading this book. Conventional treatments miss the real cause of most back trouble—they simply don't address the stress and muscle pain problem.

Most treatments also emphasize "taking it easy," "trying not to hurt yourself," or waiting for the pain to go away before resuming activity. Yet all the research and our experience with patients show that a quick return to unrestricted physical movement is the fastest and surest way to recovery.

3. We have great news about your hurting back! *Back Sense* describes a new way to treat chronic back pain that is more ef-

fective and less expensive than conventional methods and allows you to resume full activity. Its goals are to help you understand the true causes of chronic back pain, reduce your stress, and restore your life. The especially exciting part is that you can heal yourself without special treatments and without having to accept disability and the loss of your favorite pastimes. The methods we describe have already helped thousands of back pain sufferers before you. They're safe, too—low risk for almost everyone (we'll tell you how to make sure they're right for you).

We know that all of this is *very* hard to believe if you've been stuck with back pain for months or years. We were also extremely skeptical when we first heard about it. Please take a chance and read on. The news in this book can be your way out of pain.

HAPPY ENDING: ONE PATIENT'S TRUE STORY

Up until now we have been talking about chronic back pain in general. Here is the story of one man's struggle with the ailment—how he suffered and eventually got better. Your own story will be different, but you may find similarities to what you've experienced.

> *I'm in my forties now, married, a professional. I was in my early thirties when the ordeal began. I was in decent shape and enjoyed outdoor sports. While on vacation visiting my brother, I decided to try out his cross-country ski machine. The next day, when my back started to ache, I figured that the machine had overstressed my muscles. Like most of us, I had gotten backaches before. But when I returned home from vacation, the pain was worse. I got a bit anxious when the pain moved into my leg, since I thought that this might indicate a nerve problem.*
>
> *After a couple of weeks of pain I was starting to worry. Not only was the ache still there, but my toes went numb when I was walking. I went to my doctor, who looked worried herself. She sent me to see an orthopedic surgeon connected with a famous medical school. The surgeon ordered a CAT scan of my lower spine and told me to rest in bed until the results were known.*

The CAT scan report brought dismal news. I was told that I had a herniated L5-S1 disk that was causing leg pain. The specialist reassured me that "many" patients recovered without surgery—provided they rested enough and avoided reinjuring their backs. I did not find this especially reassuring. I was given anti-inflammatory drugs, muscle relaxants, painkillers, and stern instructions to be careful. I grew dizzy, nauseated, and tired from the medicine.

Out of work, and lying in bed for hours at a time, I was bored and miserable. I had plenty of time to remember all sorts of things that hadn't occurred to me in years. I recalled that my mom had been diagnosed with a "slipped disk" when I was young. I remembered that she had spent months in bed and was forced to use a bedpan. I realized that she had never fully returned to normalcy. I began to imagine life as a disabled person, and the idea filled me with dread.

Each morning, upon awakening, I tried to figure out if the pain was better or worse. There was no clear trend. Sometimes my spirits would lift for a few hours if the pain seemed less, only to crash again when it returned.

One day an idea occurred to me. Maybe a physician specializing in sports medicine might take a more optimistic and active position about my treatment. I called and made an appointment for a consult. This doctor took one look at the disk on the CAT scan and ordered me back to bed, threatening that if I did not heed his warning, I'd be "begging for surgery" in six months.

After weeks of bed rest, the pain and numbness were getting worse. I now imagined myself never being able to ride in the car or go for a simple walk around the block. Desperate, I consulted a chiropractor. Confirming the two doctors' diagnosis, the chiropractor prescribed regular spinal manipulations, ultrasound stimulation, a back brace, and ice packs. I was excited to finally have a more active plan for getting better, and I followed the chiropractor's advice religiously. Despite my hopes, it was not long before it became obvious that the pain and numbness were not really going away.

A couple of months later I began dragging myself to work, ignoring the dire warnings. I installed a bed in my office so that I could lie down most of the time. I couldn't sit for more than ten minutes and couldn't walk for more than a block. I wore a back brace, sat on special cushions, and leaned my car seat back to take the pressure off of my spine. More than once I almost got into an accident because I could hardly see through the windshield.

I now thought of little but my back and leg pain and was terrified of every movement. I became angry, depressed, and bitter. I had always hoped to have children, but I couldn't even take care of myself now. My wife was depressed and exhausted, too, after months of caring for an invalid. One day my wife got fed up with me and suggested that I seemed to complain of more pain when I was emotionally agitated. I dismissed the idea as nonsense and angrily accused her of blaming me for a condition that was beyond my control. She clearly just didn't understand.

A friend at work, hearing of my troubles, suggested that I look into the treatment methods of John Sarno, a famous doctor in New York. Dr. Sarno had supposedly helped a mutual acquaintance. Having read several medical books and seen three doctors, I felt that I already knew enough about back pain treatment to last a lifetime. I ignored the recommendation. The friend again pushed the idea a couple of months later. Fresh out of options, I gave in.

Dr. Sarno's rather strange and improbable idea was that most chronic back pain, and the associated sciatic nerve symptoms, were not due to displaced disks or other structural problems at all. Rather, he insisted, these symptoms were caused by physical reactions to emotional stress. It can't be true, I thought. The pain was too real. The CAT scan was too clear. The doctors and the books all agreed. There was that annoying observation from my wife, though, about my being in more pain when I was upset. Could there possibly be something to this guy's theory? I wondered.

I called the woman who had supposedly benefited from seeing Dr. Sarno.

"How long have you been laid up?" she asked.

"About four months," I replied.

"What are you doing now?" she asked.

"Lying down, of course—that's all I ever do."

"Why don't you go out and buy groceries for the family—your wife will appreciate it."

"Are you crazy?" I inquired.

"No—try it! I spent a year being completely crippled before figuring this out. I've been fine ever since."

I was completely stunned by this conversation. The woman was serious. As far as I knew, she wasn't insane. My situation seemed so dire, yet I wanted to believe that there was a way out.

Summoning all my courage, I decided to try walking around the block. This seemed like a major expedition after all the months of bed rest. As I progressed, filled with the familiar fear, I noticed that my sciatic pain was now moving from one leg to the other. With a sudden shock I realized that this didn't make any sense—the CAT scan clearly showed the disk protruding to one side. Only one leg should be hurting. If the pain was shifting sides, maybe it wasn't being caused by the disk after all!

The following few weeks brought about a remarkable transformation. Gradually, despite my worries, I began moving again. I started to realize that more movement did not always lead to more pain. Sometimes the pain stayed the same, or even diminished, despite the fact that I was doing things that should irritate my damaged spine. Little by little I began acting more normally.

During this time I realized that I had suffered from medical problems in the past that might have been stress-related, including a persistent "pinched nerve" in my neck and chronic heartburn. There seemed to be a pattern here.

Increasingly convinced that my back trouble was probably caused by fear and muscle tension, I started working on regaining my range of motion and rebuilding lost muscle strength. There were ups and downs. When the pain intensified, I would get very discouraged. Still, doing more helped build my confidence, and as it grew, my pain began to diminish. I trained my friends to stop asking about my back and ask instead how I was doing with my fears. My depression and anxiety lifted as prospects of a normal life returned. Over the next several months I gradually returned to the full range of activities I had enjoyed before that fateful day on the cross-country ski machine.

These events took place about ten years ago. This patient is important to us. That is not only because he was, in a sense, our first patient. It is because he is Dr. Ronald Siegel, a clinical psychologist and one of the authors of this book.

Dr. Siegel's story illustrates several crucial points about chronic back pain. Note that even the best doctors may make errors in treating the problem. They are trapped by the same misconceptions about its cause and treatment as are patients. Also, the damaged spine theory of back pain seems so powerfully sensible that we tend to believe in it, even when the facts of our own situation don't really fit. We have found that patients' first major breakthrough in treatment often occurs when they notice for themselves that their symptoms aren't entirely consistent with their diagnosis. Dr. Siegel's experience of pain shifting from one leg to the other is just one example of how this happens. His story also shows that motivated, functional people can get caught in the intense downward spiral of the chronic back pain syndrome. In addition, it demonstrates how it is common for back pain patients to have suffered from other stress-related problems in the past. These can include headaches, digestive difficulties, rashes, jaw pain, grinding teeth, neck aches, joint pain, fatigue, and insomnia. Finally, the story illustrates how chronic back pain can rob people of the athletic, social, or other pursuits that they once used to relieve stress. This, of course, only compounds the problem.

You may be thinking that this is a strange and interesting story, and these are curious ideas, but they don't apply to you. Your back really *is* damaged. Your thoughts and feelings couldn't have anything to do with your back pain. Your pain is too severe to be the result of tight muscles. The plain fact is, muscle tension can produce tremendous pain, under the right circumstances. Unbelievable as it may seem, you too can leave your back pain behind.

IS THIS BOOK FOR YOU?

The Back Sense program is suitable for almost anyone suffering from pain in the back or neck, as well as related pain that is felt in the legs or arms, that has lasted for more than a couple of months. While we use the term *back* throughout the book, the treatment principles we outline apply equally well to most neck pain. We say "almost anyone" because there are a very small number of chronic back pain cases that are caused by some kind of underlying medical problem that requires special attention. This is an exception to the rule that affects only about one in two hundred people.

Health care professionals make a distinction between *acute* and *chronic* back pain. Usually acute refers to pain lasting less than two or three months, while chronic indicates it has lasted longer. Acute back pain may be thought of as primarily a bodily problem, whereas chronic back pain involves the mind and the body. Often, acute back pain is caused by common injuries such as muscle strains. These usually heal on their own in a month or two. While the principles we will be describing can help prevent acute back pain from turning into chronic back pain, they are designed especially for people whose pain has persisted. If your pain has lasted for at least two months and doesn't seem to be getting better, you are probably getting caught in the chronic back pain syndrome caused by muscle tension.

Chronic back pain comes in many forms. Some of our patients have suffered with the problem for just a few months, while others have struggled with pain for several decades. For some it has been merely annoying, for others completely disabling.

We want to emphasize the fact that stress-related chronic back pain often *begins* with an acute physical injury. This can be due to an accident, overuse of muscles, or strain. Sometimes, however, the pain begins during an unremarkable action such as cleaning the house or playing a sport. For a surprising number of people, the pain seems to begin "out of the blue" and isn't directly connected to any single event. Even though there may not be a clear-cut event that caused the pain, people try hard to make sense of their pain and tend to search exhaustively for anything damaging that they have engaged in.

People with chronic back pain come from all walks of life. Some have worked at jobs that require physical exertion, while others have sat at desks for many years. Some have been truly athletic, while others were never unusually strong or physically fit.

The diagnoses we see are also varied. Many have been told that they have a "slipped," "bulging," "herniated," or "degenerated" disk. Others have been told that they have arthritis in the spine or that their spine is misaligned (subluxations), curved (scoliosis) or otherwise malformed, damaged, or weak. Some of our patients have been told that nothing is wrong with them physically, and they must be imagining their pain. They may have been informed that the tests "didn't find anything" or been given a diagnosis such as "idiopathic back pain," which means the same thing. Many of them are simply given pain medication, tranquilizers, or antidepressants and sent on their way. They are often left thinking that their doctor hasn't looked hard enough to find what is really wrong with them.

However your pain began, and whatever your diagnosis, chances are that your pain is not due to damage to your spine. Even the fact that tests may have shown something to be out of place or "degenerated" need not be cause for alarm. Similarly, observations about misalignment or bad posture may have nothing to do with your pain. We will show you in the pages ahead how concerns about being damaged, along with other sources of stress and tension, are enough to cause and maintain your pain. Again, this does *not* mean that the problem is just psychological. Rather, you will learn how certain beliefs and emotional attitudes can cause you to unknowingly tense muscles and how muscle tightness and spasms can cause the pain you experience.

It is important to recognize that everyone has stress and tension, and anyone can get caught in the cycle of pain, worry, and stress that causes chronic back pain. The demands of modern life subject all of us to an astounding variety of stressors. While we emphasize the role of stress in the problem, it is important to realize that we are not suggesting that you need to avoid or eliminate stress to succeed with the program. Instead we teach you ways to cope effectively with the inevitable pressures of life in our society.

Whatever your diagnosis or history, if you find yourself frustrated by your lack of progress in overcoming chronic back pain, this book is indeed for you.

WHY HASN'T MY DOCTOR TOLD ME ABOUT THIS?

At this point, alarm bells may be going off in your mind in response to all this supposedly good news. You may be thinking: *If these methods are such a "breakthrough," why doesn't my doctor know about them? He or she is pretty smart. He or she went to an excellent medical school.* We understand these questions because we would be thinking the same things. After all, people have been selling crackpot science and quack cures for years. The complete answer will resolve your concerns, but it's complicated. For that reason we address it at length in chapter 3.

The short answer is that advances in medical treatment usually take a long time to be accepted. That is often not such a bad thing. You want to be careful when you are dealing with someone's health. Luckily we are not talking about brain surgery. The risks in this case are tiny, and the conventional treatments themselves actually involve a good deal of risk. Many of them actually make things worse!

The self-treatment methods we will show you involve both the body and the mind. Most doctors simply haven't been trained to think this way. Study after study finds that chronic pain is often unrelated to the condition of the spine. Study after study also shows stress to be the most important predictor of who gets back pain. Most health professionals working with chronic pain do accept the idea that this plays *some* role in how intense the pain seems to patients. They are generally unaware, however, of the research demonstrating that the mind can be potent enough to actually cause the problem by increasing tension in the body.

MEDICINE AND ALTERNATIVE MEDICINE

In recent years there has been a rapidly growing interest in what has come to be known as *alternative medicine.* A wide variety of so-called alternative practitioners offer services to back pain sufferers, and these individuals sometimes think of themselves as working in opposition to what they call *conventional, traditional,* or *Western medicine* (others say that they are working to complement conventional medicine).

Many people have asked whether the Back Sense program is alternative medicine. The answer is complicated because the term means so many different things to different people. We have already noted that, strictly speaking, our ideas are an alternative to conventional medical understanding and treatment of chronic back pain. At the same time, as we will show you, our methods are grounded in recent, solid scientific research from around the world.

Our program, which draws upon the most useful contributions of both conventional and alternative medicine, is part of an exciting trend called *integrative medicine*. It is well suited to problems such as chronic back pain in which stress plays an important role.

The Back Sense perspective may appear to slight the physical side of back pain treatment. This is not the case. We know that primarily physical approaches *can* help.

Because chronic back pain is caused by tight muscles, any treatment that relaxes them can alleviate the pain, at least temporarily. Some health professionals who recognize that the pain is due to muscle tension call the problem *myofascial pain*. They identify specific problematic muscles. Heat, massage, manipulation, exercise, injections, and stretches can all help to relax these. This can break the cycle and lead to permanent relief. In fact, any intervention that gets people moving normally, and trusting that their back is basically intact, can bring an end to the pain.

If you are drawn to the material in this book, physical treatments alone probably haven't worked. By understanding and addressing the role of *both* the mind and the body, the Back Sense program more reliably breaks the back pain cycle.

CHAPTER 2

WHAT *IS* THE PROGRAM?

THIS CHAPTER EXPLAINS:

- **The essential elements of the self-treatment program**
- **How to use this book effectively**
- **How to analyze your understanding of back pain**

The Back Sense program is a brand-new and powerful method for helping you to recover from chronic back pain. It grew out of personal suffering and was refined through over ten years of clinical practice in psychology and medicine. While the Back Sense program requires more personal commitment than traditional treatments such as pills, injections, or spinal manipulation, the effort is rewarded by long-term results.

Before you actually begin self-treatment, we help you to get the right kind of medical evaluation to rule out the very unlikely possibility that a *truly* serious medical condition is causing your problem. *It is essential that you not skip this step.* The key here is to separate the *truly serious* from the *falsely thought to be serious.* Once this is settled, you can begin the program. At this point we want to give you a preview of what it is all about. It has only four basic parts (illustrated in figure 1):

1. Learning to understand the real causes of chronic back pain: In this part of the program we explain what is wrong with the traditional medical understanding of back pain and how we know that it is wrong. We also help you to properly understand how you developed chronic back pain in the first place and why it continues to plague you. The idea that the pain is the result of physical problems with your spine is so seemingly obvious, natural, and logical that it requires a good deal of effort to show you that it's not true. It's very important that we do this because your *beliefs* about what is wrong can actually augment the pain. Working with beliefs in this way is a central part of the most effective treatments for these sorts of stress-related problems.

2. Learning to understand your own case of chronic back pain: You probably have your own ideas about what caused your problem and what movements and circumstances make your pain better or worse. Examining these ideas and gradually modifying them as you uncover flaws are very important parts of the program. We teach you exercises that help you do just that. Beginning to see *for yourself* that your back isn't really "bad" gives you the confidence to try the physical activities that will help you to recover fully.

3. Learning to resume full physical activity: In contrast with most treatments for chronic back pain that tend to focus just on relieving your pain, the Back Sense program concentrates on helping you resume full activity and restore physical functioning. There are several reasons for this. Much of the tension-producing negative emotion surrounding chronic back pain is due to fear and frustration about not being able to live life fully. Only by returning to normalcy can these feelings be resolved. Furthermore, by proving to yourself that you can live a normal life, and even exercise vigorously,

THE BACK SENSE PROGRAM

Before Beginning the Program

- Getting a medical evaluation to rule out truly serious conditions

CHAPTER: 4

1. Learning to Understand the Real Causes of Chronic Back Pain

- The conventional medical understanding of chronic back pain—what's wrong with it and how we know
- Excellent prognosis—the new research-based understanding of how muscle tension causes chronic back pain
- Why your doctor may not know about all this

CHAPTERS: 1, 2, 3, 5, 6

2. Learning to Understand Your Own Case of Chronic Back Pain

- Exploring your personal symptoms and ideas about your pain problem
- Testing and debunking beliefs about what makes your pain problem better or worse

CHAPTER: 7

3. Learning to Resume Full Physical Activity

- Taking stock of the activities you've curtailed and limited because of back pain
- Gradually and systematically restoring a normal spectrum of physical activity
- Using mindfulness, exercise, and scientific principles to manage problems that come up in moving again

CHAPTERS: 8, 12, 13

4. Learning to Work with Negative Emotions

- How emotional reactions to your pain problem worsen the syndrome
- How emotional reactions to stressful life situations and certain styles of handling emotion worsen the syndrome
- Using insight and mindfulness to prevent negative emotions from derailing your recuperation

CHAPTERS: 9, 10, 11, 12

Figure 1

you see for yourself that there is nothing wrong with your back itself. Until you truly believe this, every occurrence of back pain will continue to cause anxiety, tension, and hence more pain. We will show you proven techniques for dealing with any temporary discomfort or worries that may arise.

Until now, you have probably been told to rest and protect your back. This often causes people to become seriously deconditioned. We teach you how to safely improve your strength, flexibility, and endurance with a range of exercises. These have a number of beneficial effects, including relieving stress, restoring normal sleep patterns, reducing fear of movement, reducing the weakness and inflexibility of muscles that can produce back pain, and "immunizing" the body against minor physical injuries.

4. Learning to work with negative emotions: If you suffer from chronic back pain, you have probably experienced fear, anger, anxiety, frustration, depression, and other similar demons in connection with it. These difficult emotions are the natural result of a seriously disabling problem. They also often play a huge role in keeping chronic back pain going by causing you to tense muscles that can directly produce the pain. Learning to detect and manage these stress states can actually help you to break out of your pain.

Each part of the program helps to support the others. While we will guide you step by step, the changes you make in one area will make it easier to tackle other parts of the program. All of your efforts will eventually come together.

THIS BOOK IS A TOOL

Getting the most out of Back Sense

We are amazed, and amused, by all the different self-help books that are out there. You may be, too, and you may have noticed that their quality varies quite a bit. You will probably not be surprised when we say that we have tried to bring you reliable information of the very highest quality. As a former landlady once remarked when we told her we were especially neat and clean, "Everybody says that!"

Many self-help books tell you about ways to solve a problem. What is different about this one is that just reading it can be a major step in actually curing chronic back pain. In fact, many people will begin to feel relief shortly after finishing it. That's because believing your pain is the result of a damaged back is in itself a major cause of the pain, and this book attacks that stubborn belief. We feel that a mostly self-treatment approach is the right one because chronic back pain is still so widely misunderstood by health care practitioners. That means there is a current shortage of professionals who can help you apply our methods.

For these reasons, we like to think of the book as a tool. With that in mind, we've tried to make it as "user-friendly" as possible. We have kept it relatively free of medical jargon (except where it can help you to better understand doctors' language). We try to deal with technical points in a way that explains them without burying you under a pile of unnecessary details. If you are skeptical, or want more information, our scientific sources are all cited in the reference section, and related books are listed in an appendix. We also include stories from the experiences of many other chronic back pain sufferers.

We offer participatory exercises throughout the book to help you. Taking the time to complete these can be beneficial, but we know that some readers prefer to read straight through without stopping. If this is your style, just read first and come back to them.

Each person suffering from chronic back pain is unique. For some the pain syndrome resolves quickly; for others it takes longer. Also, depending upon how you understand the cause of your pain, how restricted your movement has become, how disturbing the pain has been, and what other sources of stress you have in your life, some parts of this book will be more important to you than others.

It should be recognized from the start that you may not need to read all sections of *Back Sense* or complete all parts of the program to get better. If your doubts about our understanding of the problem are resolved early on, it is not necessary to continue through the first sections of the book, which establish how we know what we know about back pain and why we recommend what we do to fix it. In that case, by all means, begin resuming activities (chapter 8) and refer back to the supporting material as needed. Similarly, if you are able to make steady progress in restoring activities, feel free to gloss over our later material on the complicating emotional issues and life situations that prevent many people from becoming pain free.

Describing our major points doesn't take long. Fully explaining them, answering your sensibly skeptical questions, and helping you get better takes a little longer. The rest of the book will give you "nuts and bolts" guidance.

PERSONAL BELIEFS ABOUT PAIN

A first exercise

Because beliefs are so important in chronic back pain problems, the first step in getting well involves examining your particular ideas about the cause of your pain. Before we go further, please take a few minutes to complete the "Beliefs about Pain" exercise. This will help you to clarify your current ideas.

BELIEFS ABOUT PAIN

CAUSES OF THE PROBLEM

In the beginning, what did you think caused your pain? What made you believe this?

____

____

What have doctors and/or other professionals told you about the cause of your pain?

____

____

If you have had diagnostic tests, what did they say? Did you trust them?

____

____

Have your ideas about what causes your pain changed over time? If so, how and why?

____

____

Describe your mental picture of your back. What do you think is loose, damaged, scraping, rubbing, pinched, weak, tight, and so forth? If you think your back is deteriorating, what process is causing this?

____

____

Of the ideas you've had about your back, which have been the most upsetting?

____

____

Care of Your Back

Are you concerned that you may be causing damage if you engage in activities that cause pain? What makes you think this?

____

____

Have you had any experiences that convince you that you should "take it easy" on your back?

____

____

Do you have any friends or relatives who are limited by back pain?

____

____

Has resting your back made you feel better overall (over the long run—not just on particular days)?

____

____

Should you stop doing something if it starts to cause you pain?

Do you think you will need to permanently restrict some of your activities?

Do you worry about other people expecting you to do more than you can do?

CHAPTER

3

BAD BACK?

THIS CHAPTER EXPLAINS:

- **How the back is constructed**
- **Why chronic back pain is usually *misunderstood* to be the result of a damaged spine**
- **The overwhelming current scientific evidence that reveals that structural damage is almost always *not* the cause of the pain**
- **Why most health care professionals have been slow to realize this**

It is completely natural to assume that if your back hurts, it must be because of an injury or illness. We all learn to connect physical pain with underlying injury. When we cut our finger, we see blood and feel pain. If we bump into something hard, it hurts and a bruise appears. Often the amount of pain corresponds to the extent of the visible damage. As the damage heals, the pain diminishes. Why should back pain be any different? When our back is "killing us," we of course think something *must be* terribly wrong. You may well have been told by a doctor that you were born with an abnormal spine or that some structure in your back has deteriorated or been damaged and that those things are the cause of your problem. Most of the explanations we hear from experts reinforce such ideas, but the scientific evidence points in a completely different direction. The plain fact is that on rare occasions some sort of damage *is* a factor in chronic back pain, but usually it is not.

HOW THE BACK IS BUILT

The parts of the back and how they work

To understand our key points, it is helpful to take a quick look at the structures of the back. Some of you may have already learned more about spinal anatomy than you ever wanted to know, by seeing frightening pictures of your supposedly damaged spine at the doctor's office, looking at diagrams, or reading other books. We'll limit ourselves here to the basic facts you need.

Figure 2 illustrates the basic parts of the back. The *spine* is an extremely rugged scaffolding that supports the body. It is made of a stack of small blocks of bone called *vertebrae.* Between each vertebra is a tough, rubbery *disk* that provides cushioning and increases the flexibility of the joint. The back also includes a powerful complex of muscles. There are very short muscles that attach to the vertebrae directly and longer muscles that attach all along the spine.

There are several variants in the anatomy of the back (reviewed in more detail in appendix 1). Some of the most commonly described ones involve the disks. ***Disk bulges*** are simply protruding irregularities in the shape of the disk, while ***disk herniation*** is a deformity of the disk caused by a tear in its outer surface. Both of these are also often blamed for back pain, or ***sciatica,*** a name for pain that runs down the leg. While disk herniations can sometimes put pressure on the nerves, we will show you that disk bulges and herniations are common and are often not even noticed.

STRUCTURE OF THE SPINE

Figure 2

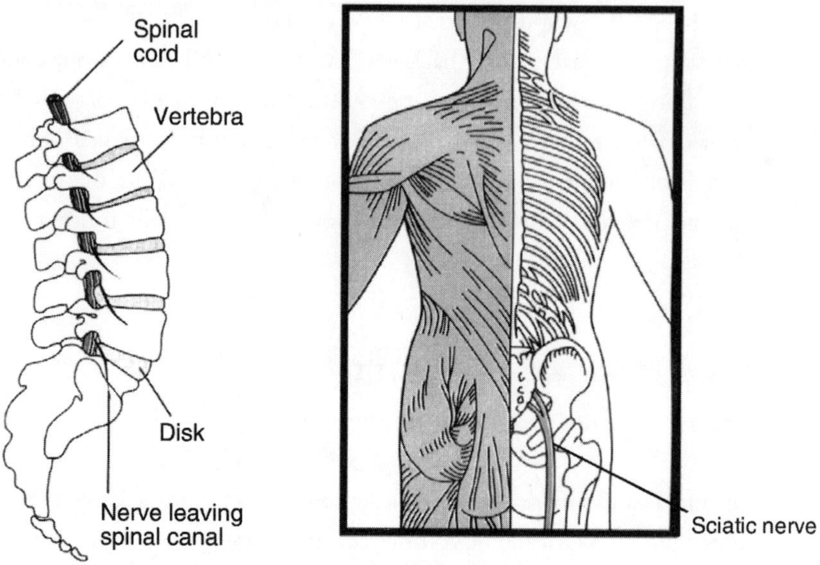

SPINAL STRUCTURE **MUSCLES OF THE BACK**

From Bigos, S., Bowyer, O., Brawyer, G., et al. *Acute Low Back Problems in Adults.* Clinical Practice Guideline No. 14. AHCPR Publication No. 95-0642. Rockville, MD: Agency for Health Care Policy and Research, Public Health Service, U.S. Department of Health and Human Services. December 1994.

THE DAMAGED BACK THEORY OF CHRONIC BACK PAIN

What most people, including physicians, believe to be the cause of chronic back pain

As should be obvious by now, the prevailing view of chronic back pain, among both patients and medical authorities, is that it is caused by some sort of damage. Unfortunately, this is presented more as "the fact of the matter" than as a theory. For this and other reasons, most people suffering from chronic back pain accept that structural damage is their primary problem. You may have been told that you had a genetic abnormality that made you vulnerable to injury; that some structure in your spine has deteriorated or been damaged; or a combination of the two. Chances are that you identified some such problem as the cause of your difficulties when you completed the "Beliefs About Pain" exercise at the end of chapter 2.

Our association between pain and structural injuries is so strong that even those people whose back pain first appears during entirely normal activity search their minds to find some event that "harmed" their back. In our work, we have repeatedly heard people say things like "It must have been from shoveling snow" two weeks before any symptoms appeared, "I think I was holding my baby the wrong way," or, "It happened vacuuming"—even though they have shoveled snow, held their baby, and vacuumed the very same way many times before. (Research shows that in reality, chronic back pain appears without any accident or injury two-thirds of the time.)

Based on their training, primary care physicians, orthopedists, neurosurgeons, chiropractors, and physical therapists generally look for some structural abnormality to explain persistent pain. Technology plays a role, too. We now have MRIs and CAT scan imaging technologies (see definitions on page 194) to show us just where the "injuries" or "defects" are. These abnormalities are each associated with a different diagnosis (the common ones are described in appendix 1). Most of these diagnoses assume that a disk or bone structure is pressing on a nerve root or, less often, that some misalignment of the body is causing the patient to stand, move, or sit in a way that chronically strains muscles, thereby producing pain. All this evidence, together with our association of pain with injury, is more than enough to convince most people that their back is damaged and that that is what is making their life miserable.

WHAT'S WRONG WITH THE DAMAGED BACK THEORY

Why we think this explanation of most chronic back pain is false

For most people, the belief that your back is damaged is abandoned only gradually. After all, sensible people don't go against common sense, personal experience, and expert medical advice without a pretty compelling set of reasons to do so.

Medical treatment is based upon science, and most of us trust medicine, at least more than anything else, when it comes to a serious pain problem. In the case of chronic back pain, scientific understanding has jumped ahead of current medical practice. Therefore, even if you are not very science minded, we encourage you to read this section carefully and follow our reasoning. It provides the solid, balanced, sensible support for almost everything we do in the Back Sense program. An absolutely essential component of the program is to start to move and act normally. This is difficult to do if you think the pain you experience means you are damaging or harming your back.

Because chronic back pain is a huge and costly public health concern, extensive research on the problem has been conducted all over the world. It has yielded pervasive scientific evidence refuting the belief that chronic back pain is caused by structural damage. The evidence can be divided into five broad categories:

1. Evidence showing that *most* people who have never suffered from serious back pain at all have the very same sorts of "damaged," "deteriorated," or "malformed" back structures that many doctors use to account for chronic back pain.

One group of studies asks the question "What exactly do 'normal' backs look like?" This is a critical issue. If it is true that structural abnormalities cause back pain, they should not be present in pain-free backs. Physicians routinely identify disk or bone structures that appear to be "out of place" in chronic back pain patients. These structures are automatically presumed to be the cause of pain, but this has proven to be false over and over again.

The key question is how common these structural "abnormalities" are in people without back pain. One illustrative study, reported in the venerable *New England Journal of Medicine,* involved MRIs that were taken of what turns out to be a very unusual group of people: those who have never had back pain for more than a couple of days in their entire life. The results were fascinating:

> *A full 64% of the pain free group had abnormal disks! Fifty-two percent had a* bulge *of some type, while 28 percent had some kind of*

herniation. *Thirty-eight percent of the subjects had an abnormality of more than one disk. In addition to disk problems, many other types of abnormal spine structures were found. Remember, these "problems" were found in people who had never suffered anything worse than a transitory backache in their lives!*

All of these frightening-sounding diagnoses are commonly presented to chronic back pain sufferers as the cause of their affliction. The authors of this landmark research concluded that such "abnormalities" when found in chronic back pain patients "may frequently be coincidental." Many other studies have produced similar conclusions.

It has become increasingly clear that many supposed "aberrations" of the spine are actually either normal variations on how people's spines are built or the result of normal wear and tear as we age. They are not signs of injury or disease.

2. Evidence indicating that many people who suffer from chronic back pain show no clear "abnormalities" in their backs whatsoever, even after extensive testing.

The second body of evidence comes from the astoundingly large group of people who are suffering from chronic back pain but whose tests come back normal:

Jane was a successful kidney specialist. After becoming an internist, she went on to acquire two additional specialties. She loved medicine and believed deeply in science.

She had suffered from mild back pain on and off throughout her many years of medical training. Since the pain had always gone away quickly, she never paid it much attention. One day her back started to hurt badly. She first tried to ignore it, but after several weeks of on-going pain, work was becoming difficult.

Jane began consulting the appropriate specialists. To her surprise, nobody could find the cause of her pain. Over the next two years she saw many orthopedists, neurologists, rheumatologists, and a physiatrist. She had CAT scans, MRIs, blood tests, and EMGs to test her nerves. They all came back normal. She had them repeated. They came back normal again. She became increasingly frustrated as her pain continued unabated despite completely normal findings on all the relevant tests conducted by the best in the business.

It turns out that Jane's story isn't unusual at all. Many patients show no abnormalities whatsoever after extensive testing. These patients typically report similar pain experiences as those with abnormal findings, including *sciatica* (radiating leg pain) and other symptoms usually attributed to structural problems of the spine. Sadly, these patients are sometimes accused of imagining or faking their pain when their spine shows absolutely no sign of disk or vertebral abnormalities. Many patients are actually disappointed when their tests come back normal, as they fear their complaints of pain will not be taken seriously or worry that the real cause of their pain is being missed.

3. Evidence demonstrating that many people with back pain who have abnormalities continue to experience their pain even after "successful" surgery to repair the problem.

The experiences of many surgery patients further call into question the link between spine "problems" and pain:

Marvin had seen many specialists for his back pain and excruciating sciatica. He had been out of work for many months. His MRI showed a herniated disk. At first the doctors proposed conservative treatment—rest and care to avoid stressing his spine—hoping that the disk would shrink back to normal on its own. Unfortunately the pain persisted, and a second MRI showed that the disk was still out of place.

The doctors proposed surgery, which he readily agreed to after months of suffering with no perceivable improvement, eager to put an end to his misery. Because of the nature of the herniation, his surgeon decided to remove the disk herniation and fuse together the vertebrae above and below it.

It took time for the fused vertebrae to grow together, but Marvin was very careful to follow all the doctor's instructions to the letter, and eventually X-rays showed that the fusion had been successful. The only problem was that Marvin's pain *was exactly the same as it had been before the operation.*

Many, many other patients recount similar stories. Surgery is very often unsuccessful as treatment for chronic back pain, even when MRIs and CAT scans show structural abnormalities. Usually the surgeries successfully remove parts of disks or modify other spinal structures. Nonetheless, sometimes the pain gets worse, sometimes it gets better, sometimes it remains the same. Regardless of the outcome, it is clear that there is no close connection between the supposedly defective spine structure and the pain.

Some fascinating results were reported by scientists who did MRIs on patients years after their surgery. In one study, over a third of the patients still had herniated disks. It turns out that the state of the disk had no bearing on whether the person continued to be in pain.

4. Evidence showing that people have often recovered from chronic back pain following an operation during which the surgeon finds absolutely nothing wrong with their backs and simply sews them up again.

Long before the invention of MRIs and CAT scans, surgeons performed exploratory back operations based upon a person's history and complaints of pain alone (if it was serious enough). Many times they cut open the back, found nothing out of place, and simply sewed up the patient again.

A major study of these cases found that almost half of the time these surgical explorations that found nothing out of place were followed by complete relief from back pain. Sciatic pain in the leg resolved following such surgeries in more than a third of the patients. It is obvious that a damaged spine was *not* the cause of pain for these patients. While the findings may shock you, researchers now understand that these individuals recovered most likely because they *believed* strongly that they were cured by the surgery. The back surgery patients were otherwise unexceptional. They were not "hypochondriacs" or especially suggestible hypnotic subjects. It turns out that mere belief is an influence on the outcome of all sorts of medical conditions and procedures. This influence is far more powerful than most people, including many doctors, realize. We will examine this more closely in the next chapter.

5. Evidence that chronic, disabling back pain occurs mostly in developed countries with high psychological stress and low physical stress.

People in developing countries frequently do all of the things that make us fear for our backs: they engage in hard physical labor, sleep on primitive mattresses, walk long distances in worn shoes, ride in uncomfortable vehicles on bumpy roads, and receive limited medical care. If chronic back pain were really due to structural damage, we would expect them to have terrible back problems.

They don't. Doctors working in these areas report that people rarely complain of back pain (in the United States, back pain is second only to colds and flu as a reason for physician visits). It is also unusual to find people in less technologically developed countries who cannot work because of their back. In fact, rates of back pain are lowest in rural areas of poor countries, where physical labor is the hardest. What is going on?

Most researchers believe that cultural differences in attitude toward back pain is the key factor. People in less developed countries treat periodic back pain as a fact of life and keep up their normal work activities. They don't fear the pain, view it as an illness, or go for medical tests. They don't rest extensively, waiting for their backs to heal. As a result, back pain tends to resolve by itself and doesn't turn into a chronic problem. If chronic back pain were actually caused by structural problems, they wouldn't be able to do this.

Let us review all the evidence we've cited here: People without pain often have "abnormal"-looking spines, while people with pain often have "normal" spines. "Successful" surgery that fixes "abnormal" structures often fails to cure chronic back pain, while surgery that does nothing at all structurally to the back often successfully relieves pain. Finally, people in developing countries, whose backs are subjected to "abuse," rarely have serious pain problems.

These findings simply make no sense at all if we continue to think that chronic back pain is due to damaged spines. Any clearheaded analysis indicates that something else *must* be the cause of the pain. The surprising truth is that almost all chronic back pain has *no relationship whatsoever* to the presence or absence of abnormal spinal structures.

We understand that this is a difficult conclusion to accept and that it takes each individual time to accept it for themselves. We don't expect you to have changed your mind about the cause of your pain after just reading about these studies. All we want is to have raised some doubt. It is more than enough for you, at this point, to be simply entertaining the idea that what we are saying *might* be true.

If you're still tempted to believe that medical diagnoses are rock solid, and that the indications for back surgery are crystal clear, consider this: Whereas one might expect the incidence of back problems to be somewhat consistent in different parts of the country, the rate at which surgeries are performed differs from one area to another. The differences aren't small, either. Some cities report an incidence of back surgery that is more than five times that of other municipalities. Similar differences occur with other types of medical procedures as well.

THE PERSISTENCE OF THE TRIED AND UNTRUE

Why many doctors continue to believe in damaged spines, in the face of all evidence to the contrary

If there is so much evidence contradicting the idea that spinal abnormalities cause chronic back pain, why do other professionals continue to focus on these things? We recognize that this is a critically important issue to address, if you are to believe what we are telling you. Given the impressive brainpower, training, and skill of the medical community, one can easily jump to the conclusion that our new program must be flawed somehow—perhaps in a way that is entirely beyond the understanding of nonexperts.

It is only sensible to have these concerns, but since trusting our methods is absolutely essential for you to feel secure in trying them, we want to take the time to explain exactly why most doctors, chiropractors, and physical therapists really *don't* know about our approach. To do that, we have to get a bit technical and describe how medical knowledge develops.

1. Outmoded methods haven't been properly tested. The plain truth is, many back pain patients recover whether or not they receive treatment, and often regardless of the type of treatment they receive. This naturally leads many doctors to feel that their treatments are successful.

Surprisingly, simply *thinking* that we will be helped by a treatment can make us feel better. This is called a *placebo effect.* While the term *placebo* is often misunderstood to refer exclusively to "fake" pills, the concept is actually quite a bit more general. The term can refer to any treatment that is presented to patients as if it were expected to be curative.

To evaluate drugs, scientists give placebo sugar pills to some patients and the real medication to others. They then compare the response of both groups to see if the drug works any better than a sugar pill. Very often both the sugar pill and the real medication bring relief!

For most conventional back pain treatments, and especially for surgery, few studies ever actually compare the treatment that is being tested to an alternative placebo treatment. This means that when most back pain treatments appear to work, there is no way to tell if patients got better because they *believed* that they received an effective treatment or because the treatment itself actually *was* effective.

2. Medical science has often ignored the power of the mind to affect the body. The idea that the mind and body have great influence on each other first fell out of favor during the 1500s. Scientists of the time began to think of the body as a sort of machine. If something goes wrong, it is because part of the apparatus is broken.

Some doctors still assume that the mind is incapable of affecting bodily processes. Because modern medicine has made astounding progress in treating diseases and injuries, this assumption has not been seriously challenged until recently. Health professionals therefore tend to look for mechanical abnormalities of the back, then look for ways to repair them. The understanding of chronic back pain that grows out of current research involves both the body and the mind. Relatively few doctors have had training in this area.

3. Science is influenced by human nature Many people have the impression that science is completely objective. In reality, science and medicine are very human enterprises. The questions scientists ask and the way results are interpreted are influenced by their personalities, politics, training, philosophies, and sources of funding.

The tentative understandings of a problem that scientists work with are often referred to as *theories* or *models.* The assumption that chronic back pain must be caused by a damaged spine is such a theory. The fact that professionals continue relying on it, despite evidence to the contrary, is hardly unique. For instance, the idea that chocolate causes acne was discredited by research done in the 1950s, but it persisted in the minds of many doctors and patients long afterward. Likewise, the idea that stomach ulcers are caused in part by bacteria and can be treated effectively with antibiotics was first ridiculed, then resisted, and finally accepted by scientists. Despite this fact, recent data suggests that some practitioners still don't prescribe antibiotic treatment.

Science usually advances slowly. The prevailing theory in a scientific field is generally not abandoned until an *overwhelming* quantity of evidence accumulates that is inconsistent with it. Until that time, even what eventually turn out to be vastly superior theories are often slighted. It also often simply takes time for new knowledge or treatments to trickle down to a majority of practitioners in the field.

Patients often wrongly assume there is a complete consensus among medical authorities about how to treat a particular problem. Even when it is true, an individual doctor may not practice in accord with that consensus. A study of official treatment guidelines found that a significant number of doctors either rejected a cookbook approach or disagreed with some of the standardized recommendations.

Despite the factors keeping doctors from embracing a new understanding of chronic back pain, a consultation with a physician is essential prior to beginning the Back Sense program. Shortly, we will present a model of chronic back pain that makes much better sense, in light of new knowledge, than conventional theories. To entertain this explanation, you'll need to feel secure that you do not have one of the rare medical causes of back pain we've alluded to.

CHAPTER 4

RULING OUT TRULY SERIOUS MEDICAL CONDITIONS

THIS CHAPTER EXPLAINS:

- **The importance of getting a good medical evaluation**
- **Where to get more information**

As we have said, there is compelling evidence that the vast majority of chronic back pain is due primarily to muscle tension and physical deconditioning. This is true even for people who experience frequent, terrible pain and have been disabled by it for many years. Nonetheless, we have alluded to the fact that there *are* exceptions to this. These include cases of tumors, infections, inflammatory diseases, and some structural injuries or malformations. Remember, these unusual problems represent only about *one-half of 1 percent* of people with back pain. Because believing they are structurally damaged can be so very harmful to all other people, we do not emphasize these other causes of back pain.

SCREENING FOR RARE PROBLEMS

Ensuring that you do not have a significant structural problem or disease

It is *crucial* that people with chronic back pain consult a physician prior to beginning to adopt the self-treatment and other methods that we advocate. This is vital for several reasons:

- **Obviously, in the unlikely possibility that you *do* have a serious and treatable medical condition, you would want to identify it and receive appropriate medical attention.**

- **You need a competent medical consultation to allow you to begin to seriously entertain the notion that your chronic pain is *not* due to structural causes. Unless you can do this, it is very difficult to begin the recovery process.**

- **You need to consult a physician to obtain permission to exercise without limitations.**

Fortunately, well-trained physicians, understanding the principles we have outlined, can definitively rule out the vast majority of serious medical disorders with a good medical work-up. Most people with chronic back pain who have access to medical care will undergo extensive medical evaluations in the course of coping with the problem. It is unlikely that these evaluations would miss one of these rare causes of pain. It is much more likely, unfortunately, that at least one of these evaluations will *mistakenly* identify some harmless structural variation, postural habit, or physical action as the primary cause of the pain.

Most physicians and other health care providers persist in pointing to abnormalities of the spine to explain chronic back pain, despite all evidence to the contrary. It can be hard to dismiss mistaken advice without an alternative *professional* opinion. At times it can be difficult to find a physician who will support your progress by encouraging unrestricted movement. If you are having difficulty, try to find a *physiatrist* (physician specializing in rehabilitation) in your area. They have special training in muscle problems and are more likely to encourage you to exercise. You can get a referral from your health care provider or obtain a list of physiatrists in your area from the American Academy of Physical Medicine and Rehabilitation (see appendix 3).

WHAT YOUR DOCTOR SHOULD LOOK FOR

The most common warning signs of serious injury or disease

Everyone feels nervous when going to the doctor for an evaluation. Nonetheless, most back pain involves muscles and isn't dangerous. Medical research is very clear that having back pain does not, in itself, mean not being able to function. It is safe to lift, bend, carry, squat, play, have sex, and participate in sports if you are one of the people without a serious medical cause of pain.

You may find it comforting to know that the government recently published a set of guidelines for diagnosing and treating back pain. It is based on a comprehensive review and analysis of all current research on the subject. For acute back pain (lasting less than one month), physicians are advised to look for so-called red flags—features of the case that suggest a greater likelihood of serious underlying problems. These may also indicate serious disease for an individual with chronic pain.

The warning signs include the following:

- **Unexplained weight loss, fevers, or chills**

- **A patient age of less than twenty or more than fifty (though muscular back pain, which is not dangerous, is also common in people in these age ranges)**

- **Recent urinary tract or other bacterial infection**
- **IV drug abuse**
- **Immune suppression from HIV, transplant, or steroids**
- **Pain that worsens when lying down, or severe nighttime pain**
- **Recent major injury (or, in an elderly patient with osteoporosis, minor injury or even strenuous lifting)**
- **A history of cancer**
- **Numbness in the groin or buttocks region**
- **Newly developed inability to urinate, incontinence, or increased frequency of urination**
- **Difficulty controlling bowel functions**
- **Extreme weakness in the legs or weakness that is rapidly becoming worse**

These red flags indicate only that there *may* be more serious disease and that further investigation is needed. If you do have any of these symptoms it is important to discuss them with your doctor.

If your doctor gave you a diagnosis that you are concerned about, we invite you to look for it in appendix 1, "Medical Diagnosis of Back Pain." This resource will help you to differentiate between the common frightening-sounding diagnoses that have little real meaning and rare diagnoses that require special treatment or restrictions.

If you have questions about an evaluation from a physician, we encourage you to look at the sections "Health History," "Physical Exam," and "Diagnostic Tests" in appendix 1. They will help you to decide whether or not you need to seek further evaluation.

If your doctor has recommended a course of treatment, we suggest you look for it in appendix 2, "Medical Treatment of Back Pain." This will help you to evaluate the pros and cons of continuing on your current course.

In addition to getting the right diagnosis, you need to seek permission to exercise without restriction. We provide suggestions for discussing this with your doctor in chapter 13, along with exercise instructions.

Many people waste months and years, going from specialist to specialist, seeking the "real" cause of their pain. They try treatment after treatment and collect a confusing tangle of ideas about what is wrong. Once you have had a through evaluation to rule out serious diseases and disorders, it may well be time to stop gathering additional opinions.

CHAPTER
5

MIND *AND* BODY IN CHRONIC BACK PAIN

THIS CHAPTER EXPLAINS:

- How your pain—even if severe—may actually be caused by stress
- How research has shown that job dissatisfaction and other stressors are closely associated with chronic back pain
- The powerful effects of stress
- The surprising ways that beliefs affect the body

We have presented evidence that most chronic back pain is not caused by a damaged spine and are assuming that you have had a medical evaluation to rule out a rare medical disorder as the cause. In order to feel assured that your back isn't damaged, you'll need a good alternate explanation. We understand that the idea that it is caused by *stress* is pretty hard to believe at first. As it turns out, scientists are learning that stress is able to cause a host of dramatic physical problems. In this chapter we want to help you to understand some of the extraordinary ways that the mind can affect the body.

YOU'VE GOT TO BE JOKING

Why it can be so hard to accept that stress causes back pain

For some people, the news that back pain isn't caused by a damaged spine is a great relief. After all, who likes surgery, bed rest, taking medicines, or paying stacks of medical bills? Nonetheless, when many other people first hear us say that their chronic pain may have a psychological component, they are unhappy or even angry:

> *After many unsuccessful attempts to get treatment for her chronic back pain and sciatica, Susan was sent by her doctor to see Dr. Siegel. She said that the referral had surprised her, because she didn't see how a psychologist could help. Still, she seemed very receptive to new ideas in the first meeting and identified many ways in which her back pain ordeal had caused her tremendous emotional stress. She was quite aware that she was often tense and unhappy about the pain and frequently despaired about ever getting better.*
>
> *During her second visit, Susan was more reserved. When asked what she was thinking, she suddenly began to cry, saying that she just couldn't believe that she could be* imagining *all of her pain. Further conversation revealed that she had been worrying all week that her doctor thought she was crazy. She had begun to doubt her own sanity.*

Susan's experience is not unusual. Often people suspect that we are saying that they have some sort of mental illness. They feel as though they are being accused of faking or imagining their pain. Previously they thought that they were injured; now they feel that we are telling them they're emotionally unbalanced. This situation is made worse by the way society accepts physical illnesses as being outside of one's control, while stigmatizing psychological or emotional problems as a sign of weakness. Simply put, nobody wants to think that they are having a "psychological problem."

Many people we see have felt dismissed by their doctors when nothing abnormal showed up on tests. Indeed, lacking a structural problem to explain the pain, it's not unusual to hear physicians say, "It must be psychological"—meaning imagined or exaggerated—and perhaps prescribe something for anxiety or depression. This can be even more upsetting than being told that something is wrong with your spine.

We therefore want to repeat that *we are not in any way suggesting that chronic back pain is fake, imaginary, an illusion, invented, or all in your head.* We are simply saying that, just like other physical disorders that have psychological roots, most chronic back pain is caused by the body's natural response to excessive stress. This response includes muscle tension, and this can produce an amazing variety of authentic problems.

A second crucial obstacle to getting better that most chronic back pain patients face is their difficulty believing that stress could be *potent* enough to cause disabling pain. Research results can be convincing here.

A study that looked at an ordinary group of people without back problems, and waited long enough to see which ones became disabled by back pain, was performed at the Boeing Aircraft Company. The investigators wanted to figure out what actually caused chronic back pain.

> *Over three thousand employees at Boeing were followed over a period of four years. Of the original group, almost three hundred employees developed disabling back pain during this period. The investigators found that psychological stress from a variety of sources predicted back pain problems more than* any *physical measure such as strength, flexibility, height, weight, or the results of physical examinations. Psychological stress was also much more important than how physically demanding their job was.*

Numerous other studies have identified dissatisfaction, stress, and lack of support at work to be causes of disabling back pain. These studies have involved thousands of people in all lines of work, from all over the developed world. Other stressors, such as the daily challenge of raising children, or working in a war zone, have also been shown to lead to significant back pain. Watching our patients recover from chronic back pain, once they understand what really causes it, further convinces us that stress is the culprit.

You may still be thinking that something was wrong with these studies. Perhaps your situation is different? To overcome these doubts, it will be essential to understand more about what stress is and how it affects our bodies.

THE STRESS RESPONSE

How a wonderful biological mechanism goes awry

We often hear friends, family, co-workers, doctors, and the media talking about "stress"—usually in the context of how it feels bad or isn't good for us. We get the clear impression that stress levels are increasing in our society. "Stressed out" has become a common answer to the everyday question "How are you?" But what exactly is stress?

It turns out that human beings share with other animals a set of physical reactions to danger that scientists call the *fight-or-flight response.* In the presence of a threat, our heart beats faster, we become more alert, and our muscles tense, as necessary preparation for taking action. It is this arousal of the mind and body that we refer to as stress. While this system works magnificently to protect us from peril, it can also be too frequently activated in a way that causes all sorts of problems.

We feel this system at work whenever we are startled or angry:

You're walking down a dark street at night. You find yourself thinking about a mugging in the neighborhood that you heard about. You hear a noise behind you. Your heart starts to beat quickly, your breathing picks up, the hair on the back of your neck is standing up. You start walking more quickly, when suddenly you hear a thud next to you, and jump, ready to either run away or defend yourself. It is the neighbor's cat.

This fight-or-flight reaction is extremely well suited to handle short-term emergencies. The changes it brings about prepare us to take immediate action in a faster, more forceful, and more effective way than we otherwise could.

Unfortunately, we tend to have the exact same emergency reactions to all sorts of nonemergencies. Two people sitting at a table pushing little wooden objects around can experience a full-blown fight-or-flight response—if the wooden objects are chess pieces and they are in the middle of a tournament. Just moving a pen across a piece of paper can put your body in an uproar if you're signing to buy a house or get a divorce. All we need to do is think about having an argument with our boss, being insulted, seeing a loved one hurt, or losing a competition, and our fight-or-flight reaction can swing into full gear.

We are often visited with anticipatory thoughts about things that *may* go wrong and retrospective thoughts about things we feel *did* go wrong. We worry about our physical well-being, with concerns about accidents, violence, financial mishaps, and disease (including fears of unremitting chronic back pain). Emotionally we have concerns about loneliness, feelings of failure or inadequacy, and worries about our work and loved ones. All manner of things can get us frustrated or angry. These normal human experiences all evoke fight-or-flight reactions of varying intensities.

THE DISTRESSING POWER OF STRESS

How our bodies respond over time

For many years physicians and medical researchers paid little attention to the long-term effects that stress might have on the body. Stress responses are often caused by emotional events, and medicine has tended to think of the emotions as relatively unimportant for treating disease.

Gradually, however, conventional medical practitioners are beginning to pay attention. Many teaching hospitals now have departments of *behavioral medicine,* which study the effects of excessive stress responses on a host of health problems.

Dan was a busy engineer with two small children. As a young man, he had occasional digestive difficulties—bloating, constipation, and heartburn—but they never lasted very long. Then a host of stomach and intestinal symptoms came on with a vengeance. And this time they just wouldn't go away. After his regular doctor couldn't help, he consulted a couple of specialists. None of the doctors found anything at all that would explain his problems. They gave him one medicine to keep his stomach from producing too much acid, another to keep his intestines from cramping, and a third to absorb gas. None of them did much to help.

As time went on, Dan became more and more anxious about his stomach. Every time he experienced discomfort after eating a certain food, he'd eliminate it from his diet. This went on and on, with his bowels only becoming increasingly disturbed as his diet became seriously restricted.

Eventually he was told by one of the specialists that the problem might be stress-related. He was encouraged to seek psychological counseling.

Dan only reluctantly followed the suggestion. While it took some time for him to believe that stress actually was causing his entire digestive system to go haywire, he eventually understood. He gradually started adding foods back into his diet, paying attention to sources of stress rather than to what he was eating. After a couple of months his system started working right again.

We and our colleagues see people like Dan all the time. Sometimes they're having digestive troubles. Other times it's headaches, insomnia, skin problems, or pain of various sorts. If their doctors can recognize that stress is affecting the problem, and if the patient can believe them, there's a good chance that they'll recover, no matter what the difficulty is.

Researchers are learning that stress responses can cause or influence an incredible range of conditions. It turns out that stress responses can raise cholesterol levels, play a role in heart disease, and even cause heart attacks. They can contribute to gastritis, ulcers, irritable bowel syndrome, and a slew of other digestive problems. Many skin problems such as eczema and acne are made worse by chronic stress. Sexual problems of every type, including impotence, premature ejaculation, and loss of sexual interest can be caused by stress. Headaches are often brought on by stress (and, like back pain, can be extremely painful even though they are harmless). Dizziness, ringing in the ears (tinnitus), asthma, and the pain from rheumatoid arthritis are made worse by stress.

Stress can also negatively affect fertility; and it actually makes surgical wounds heal more slowly. We are much more likely to catch colds and develop other infections when under stress. There is even a surprisingly strong relationship between feeling emotionally supported (which reduces stress) and surviving cancer. Stress also can lead to panic attacks, general anxiety, fatigue, difficulty concentrating, and depression. It can make mental illnesses worse. Most important for our discussion, stress causes muscle tension, which in turn can produce pains of all types, including jaw pain, neck aches, elbow pain, foot pain, knee pain, abdominal or pelvic pain, sciatica, and, of course, chronic back pain.

As you might expect, single episodes of short-term stress don't generally cause these difficulties. The trouble starts when our fight-or-flight reaction doesn't turn off. A continuous stress response, even at a low level, becomes very taxing to the body. This is what causes most chronic back pain as well as other stress-related health problems.

It is important to realize that you don't have to be in a war, or to be emotionally disturbed, for stress to cause you difficulty. The maladies we've been describing are an epidemic in modern society—they are the reason for *most* doctors visits. Almost everyone has troubles with an overactive fight-or-flight response at some point in their lives. Our eventual goal is to help you recognize and manage stress, to diffuse its effects on the body.

THE REMARKABLE POWER OF BELIEF

How the body reacts to the mind

We have said that changing your beliefs about the cause of your pain is essential. One reason for this is that our attitudes influence our choices, and, in this case, changing your beliefs will help you to resume normal activity. The other reason is that what we *believe* to be happening in our body has a dramatic effect on our stress level, our experience of pain, and hundreds of other processes.

We've discussed the way placebo effects can make it difficult to know if a treatment really works. When hearing about placebo effects, people often assume that belief might influence what people *think* is happening to them. But it can actually alter the functioning of body organs, too! There are many dramatic examples of how beliefs change the body's physiology:

> *A woman was suffering agonizing nausea and vomiting during pregnancy. Nothing the doctors could do seemed to help. Her stomach activity was measured, and it was disrupted in a way typical of severe nausea. The doctors eventually gave her a "new and very effective drug" that they promised would stop the nausea. Within twenty minutes she reported that the nausea was better, and her stomach contractions were indeed more normal. The drug the doctors had given her was actually syrup of ipecac, a medication widely used to* induce *vomiting!*

Another good example can be found in a study of individuals who received relaxation training to lower blood pressure. Half were told that their blood pressure would decline after the first session, while the other half were told that the effects would be delayed until at least after the third session. Those expecting an immediate result had, on average, a seven times greater reduction in blood pressure after the first session than those told to expect a delay.

One fact is centrally important for understanding your back pain: Beliefs, particularly in the form of expectations, have *by far* their strongest effects on our experience of pain and discomfort. Hundreds of research studies confirm that how much pain we feel from a disease or injury depends upon our expectations.

Placebos of all sorts can be very effective in raising expectations and thus relieving pain. The most powerful type of placebo isn't a pill, but surgery and other physical treatments that bring relief by making patients *believe* that they have been fixed.

> *During the 1950s an operation was often performed to eliminate chest pain due to heart problems (*angina*). This operation tied off an important artery in order to help the heart grow new blood vessels. While the surgery generally brought good results, some doctors began to doubt that it was actually increasing the heart's blood supply.*
>
> *Research was conducted to test the effectiveness of the operation. Half of the patients received the actual procedure, while the other half were only told that they were receiving it (and given skin incisions only). The beneficial effects of the skin incisions were found to be as great as that of the real surgery. The patients could exercise more, needed less medication, and reported less chest pain because they* thought *that the surgery had fixed their problem.*

A less extreme placebo treatment was able to cure *TMJ* (*temporomandibular disorder*), a form of chronic jaw and facial pain. In this study, dentists told patients that they were going to treat their problem by grinding their teeth to improve their bite. They then put the patients through a procedure made to feel like tooth grinding, that didn't actually remove any enamel from their teeth. Even though the sham procedure did nothing real to their mouths, 64 percent of patients reported total or near total relief.

Placebos even appear to "create" side effects. Patients often report drowsiness, headaches, nervousness, insomnia, nausea, and constipation after taking a placebo pill. These reactions are much *more* common when people are warned in advance of negative effects.

Most people are surprised to learn just how substantial and wide-ranging the effects of placebos are. We may think that they must affect only very suggestible people or those with emotional problems. Actually there is *no* clear pattern whatsoever as to what sort of person will have the strongest response to placebos. The very same individual may respond more strongly in one situation than in another. Research shows that what matters most is how much a person trusts the one who offers the placebo or suggestion, and the enthusiasm of the offerer.

Research also shows that we are most likely to respond to placebos when we are anxious. As we become increasingly apprehensive about our chronic back pain, our tension and pain levels are more influenced by our expectations.

The important point is that *almost everyone's* body responds to belief to some degree, and often very powerfully. The power of belief explains why so many different back pain treatments, even when based on completely contradictory theories, are *sometimes* effective. It also explains why new treatments that often look so promising when pioneered by their enthusiastic inventor fail to live up to that promise in the long run.

Where chronic back pain is concerned, there are excellent reasons to infer that placebo effects may be responsible for the success of many surgeries, injections, chiropractic treatments, acupuncture, bracelets, magnets, special chairs, braces, and other remedies. These may all relieve back pain through their effect on the *mind,* which affects back muscles. You may come to find that this explains why you once found a certain treatment to be effective, though it no longer seems to work. Understanding this will be very useful as you move forward.

For many disorders, we do not actually know the mechanisms by which the mind influences the body. In the case of chronic back pain, however, we think that there are sound explanations, with good evidence to support them, for how stress produces and perpetuates pain. We will show you in the next chapter how this works.

CHAPTER

6

THE CHRONIC BACK PAIN CYCLE

THIS CHAPTER EXPLAINS:

- **How stress creates muscle tension and muscle tension creates pain**
- **How believing that your back is damaged can trap you in a vicious pain cycle**
- **The ways that psychological conditioning deceives us into fearing activity**
- **How frustration, anger, and depression can deepen the cycle**

We've seen so far that there isn't much relationship at all between apparent "damage" to the spine and chronic back pain. Many people with no pain have structures out of place, while other people with chronic pain seem to have nothing wrong with their spines at all. Then there are all of the people whose surgery "successfully" repaired a problem, but their pain is still there; and others whose surgery seemed to leave problems unrepaired, but the pain is gone. We've also seen that stress can have very powerful effects on the body, and it can cause a surprising number of medical problems. On top of this, it turns out that what we *believe* is happening to us physically dramatically influences both our perception of pain and our physiology.

We will now bring all this information together to show you how the effects of stress and belief combine to cause most chronic back pain.

UNDERSTANDING STRESS, FEAR, AND MUSCLE TENSION

The primary elements of chronic back pain

Recall that an important element of the fight-or-flight response is increased muscle tension. So how can this tension cause chronic back pain? Many of our patients point out that their pain doesn't *feel* like tightness or tension—it really hurts! Actually, if muscles become tense enough, or remain tense long enough, they can hurt quite a bit. If you've ever had a cramp in your calf muscle or foot, you know that these can be excruciating, making it impossible to walk until they're gone. Another example is the intense pain that comes from abdominal cramps, whether associated with indigestion or with menstruation. The interesting thing is that we generally remain largely unconcerned about these incidents of muscle tension, even if they hurt a lot. We think of them as harmless and expect them to pass before long.

Recall, too, that a host of social and emotional situations can cause stress. Psychological stress and physical muscle tension are probably best understood as two sides of the same coin. In English we use the same word, *tense,* to describe both emotional stress and muscle tension (other languages are similar). Many people notice that after a hard day at work or conflicts at home, their shoulders and neck muscles have become tight.

It is also no accident that some of the most commonly used muscle relaxants in medicine are the *benzodiazepines,* such as Valium, Ativan, and Xanax. These drugs are also widely prescribed as tranquilizers, given to help people relax or relieve anxiety. Similarly, most people find that things that relax muscles, such as exercise, massage, or sitting in a hot tub, also reduce psychological stress and lead to mental relaxation and peaceful emotions.

THE CYCLE OF CHRONIC BACK PAIN

How pain, negative thoughts, and fear interact to maintain chronic back pain

You may find it helpful at this point to look at figure 3, "The Chronic Back Pain Cycle." It shows how chronic back pain is part of a chain of events, in which one leads to another.

Chronic back pain can begin with an event that is primarily physical in nature. Physical events include the wide variety of injuries that can cause acute (short-lived) back pain. For example, you may have strained or "pulled" a muscle by lifting an unusually heavy object:

> *Nancy was hurrying to get her two-year-old son to daycare so that she wouldn't be late for work. When they arrived at the daycare center, he refused to get out of the car. She didn't have time to negotiate, so she reached in, unbuckled his car seat, and lifted him out. At that moment she felt a "pop" in her back and a stab of pain on her left side. The pain was intense, but she managed to get her son inside. By the end of the day, however, her lower back was throbbing. She couldn't find a comfortable position. Pain was shooting down her leg, and she began to get scared.*

Perhaps, instead, your acute back pain began with overusing muscles, engaging in exercise that was beyond your body's level of physical conditioning at the time:

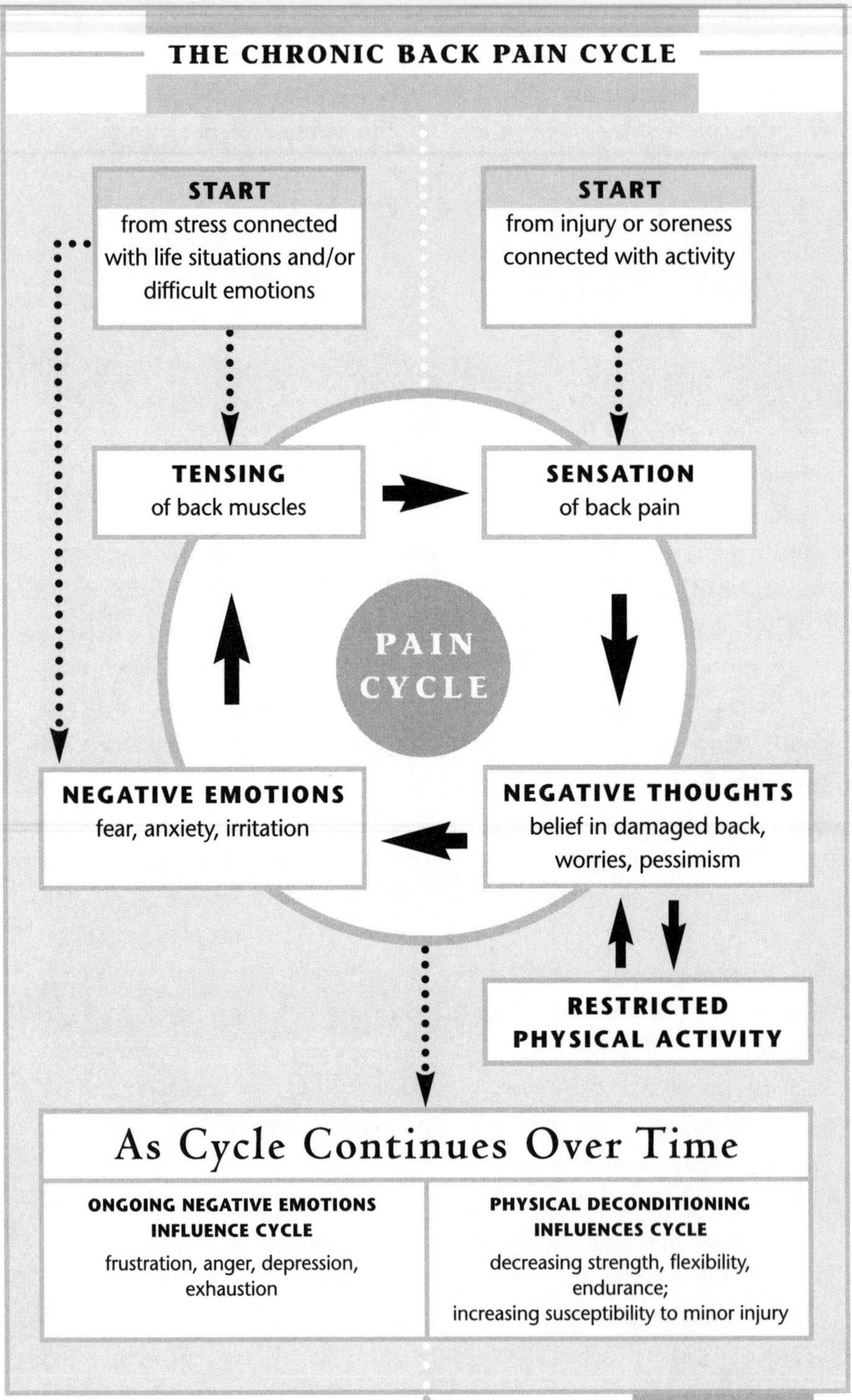
THE CHRONIC BACK PAIN CYCLE
START
from stress connected with life situations and/or difficult emotions
START
from injury or soreness connected with activity
TENSING
of back muscles
SENSATION
of back pain
PAIN CYCLE
NEGATIVE EMOTIONS
fear, anxiety, irritation
NEGATIVE THOUGHTS
belief in damaged back, worries, pessimism
RESTRICTED PHYSICAL ACTIVITY
As Cycle Continues Over Time
ONGOING NEGATIVE EMOTIONS INFLUENCE CYCLE
frustration, anger, depression, exhaustion
PHYSICAL DECONDITIONING INFLUENCES CYCLE
decreasing strength, flexibility, endurance;
increasing susceptibility to minor injury

Figure 3

Merrill knows *how his pain began. It had been a warm winter, with little snow. That all changed in January, when a big blizzard hit. He hadn't been exercising much, but the driveway needed shoveling. Though the snow was wet and heavy, he wanted to finish the job.*

The next morning he was in agony. He could barely get out of bed. He had to call in sick at work.

Acute back pain can also often begin with a fall or other accident that causes trauma to some part of the back.

While it may surprise you, the truth is that it is not too important what physical event may have caused your pain to begin. The vast majority of *acute* back pain episodes heal themselves within a month or two without any special treatment. When they don't, both patients and doctors usually start to get apprehensive about underlying structural damage to the spine. As we saw earlier, something is often found, for spinal "abnormalities" are extremely common in the general population.

Whether or not one of these "abnormalities" was found, it is very likely that your acute back injury *has* already healed. If you are still hurting after a couple of months, chances are that psychological stress has transformed your acute back injuries into a chronic muscle tension problem that is now causing your pain.

Sometimes the stress involves pressures at work or financial concerns. Other times it is caused by trouble in relationships. For many people, the stress involves difficulty managing uncomfortable emotions, such as anger or sexual feelings. Sometimes we know the sources of our stress. Other times we just feel a sense of tension, being "wound up," general unhappiness, or a lack of interest or energy for life.

For many of our patients, their greatest single source of psychological stress quickly becomes worry and aggravation about their back pain itself. As you probably know all too well, back trouble can interfere with an astounding number of activities. Once our back muscles start hurting, we suddenly notice that we use them in almost everything we do. Sitting, walking, standing, and traveling in a vehicle can all become extremely painful.

At some point, most people with chronic back pain become upset about it. Some will say that they are worried, anxious, or frightened;

others talk more about being aggravated, angry, or frustrated. If the pain has lasted a long time, people often feel depressed or hopeless. Our particular pain history and personal circumstances both influence how we feel about it. Sometimes an episode is extremely painful, and we fear having to go through it again. Other times we fear being disabled or unable to work and earn a living, take care of children, maintain relationships, or pursue our interests. We may be frustrated or angry with doctors who were unable to help. Regardless of their specific content, the impact of these feelings on the chronic back pain cycle is remarkably similar.

So here is how the chronic back pain cycle works: It may begin with a physical injury such as a pulled muscle, overexercising, or an accident. Then we become anxious or upset about our back pain, which makes the muscles of our backs tense. This, of course, only increases our pain level. Soon a vicious cycle gets going in which our pain causes emotional stress, which causes our muscles to tighten further. This in turn causes more pain, which causes more emotional stress, which leads to yet more pain. Along the way, we usually become afraid to use our back normally, which causes our muscles to become tighter, weaker, and more painful. This cycle can last for days, weeks, and even years. It can persist long after the original injury has healed.

WHAT IF I NEVER HAD AN INJURY?

For many people, back pain starts without any identifiable trauma, unusual movements, or strenuous events preceding it whatsoever. People will often think that they were hurt by something rather implausible, such as picking up a pencil the "wrong way," sleeping on a "bad" mattress, or driving a new car. We will often blame the pain on things that we did days or even weeks before:

> *Mary's lower back pain began as morning stiffness, but gradually progressed to all-day stiffness and sharp, stabbing pains. Despite this slow, incremental onset, Mary thought that she must have done* something *to cause it. It was a mystery—the pain had begun at a time when she had almost no time for physical exertion. After giving*

it a lot of thought, she decided that her problem had been caused by raking leaves, even though her first symptoms didn't appear until a full two weeks after she had finished cleaning up her yard.

While overworking muscles can cause pain, it should have appeared within the next day or two and would have resolved within two weeks. For Mary, as well as many other people without an obvious physical cause for their pain, it is far more likely that emotional stress brought on the pain.

When we are under psychological stress, our muscles become tense. Eventually, this tension leads either to muscle spasms which are intensely painful, or dull aches. When such back pain persists, we become aggravated about it, usually because we become frightened of the pain itself or the possibility of disability. We may also become frustrated or angry. These feelings further tighten the muscles, lead to more pain, and the cycle is off and running.

BUT I DON'T FEEL THAT UPSET—I DON'T THINK THIS COULD APPLY TO ME

People vary tremendously in how readily they notice signs of stress or emotional discomfort. For some, the slightest change in mood or feeling is completely apparent; for others, noticing upset appears to require a major event. The important thing to understand is that it is not at all unusual for our body to react to emotional stress that we're completely unaware of.

Even very mild emotional reactions can be seen quite clearly in the body if we use sufficiently sensitive instruments. Most of us have seen lie detectors being used on TV. These machines measure stress-related changes in vital signs, like blood pressure, to detect lying. The person being tested often doesn't notice his or her own stress responses, but they can be readily measured by the equipment.

This often explains why back pain and other tension-related problems, seem to come upon us "from nowhere." Actually, scientists have proven that we are much more likely to suffer from these sorts of problems if emotionally charged events have happened to us in recent months. Our symptoms seem to come from nowhere, either because we don't notice our emotional reactions to events in our lives or because we don't perceive the connection between our emotions and our symptoms.

Some very interesting discoveries have been made by researchers in studying the role of emotional reactions in chronic back pain. Their work is very important, because it demonstrates directly how our distress about back pain actually causes muscle tension.

The scientists selected a group of people who had been suffering from chronic back pain for more than six months and a group without back pain. The chronic back pain patients had a wide range of diagnoses.

The investigators used a machine to measure muscle tension in the back. They then tested the people's responses to different situations designed to provoke varying stress reactions. Some situations were nonstressful, while others involved recalling upsetting life events and recent bouts of pain.

While the back muscle tension of people without back pain varied somewhat during these activities, the variations were small. The dramatic finding was that chronic back pain patients, in particular, showed significantly *increased back muscle tension* when talking about emotionally loaded events. Interestingly, when the investigators measured tension in another muscle group often impacted by stress (the forehead), they found no significant differences between the back pain patients and the others.

These results suggest that for people with chronic back pain, back muscles tighten when emotionally distraught, including when thinking about pain episodes. People without chronic back pain do not tighten their back muscles to the same degree when upset. Research also shows that people with pain in other body areas, such as the jaw, specifically tense *those* muscles when they are upset.

In line with this research, we've seen countless examples of patients noticing that their back muscles tense and pain increases when they're dealing with emotional stress. Remember, Dr. Siegel's wife noticed that he complained more of pain after arguments. Later, when he was recovering, he would notice his pain recurring whenever he was asked about his disk.

A TOXIC IDEA

How faith in the damaged back theory makes chronic back pain even worse

For most people, the idea that their back is damaged is *itself* a major contributor to the cycle of pain, distress, and tension. Believing that our back is defective leads us both to experience unnecessary fear and to avoid anything that we associate with pain.

Many patients tell us that they continuously watch their pain level to figure out which things they do may be injuring them. They become anxious about walking, lifting, sitting, standing, twisting, or bending "too much" or the "wrong way." They become afraid to "irritate a nerve," "cause inflammation," "reinjure the disk," or otherwise exacerbate what they believe to be the structural cause of their pain. You, too, may find your mind full of concerns about having the right bed, chair, automobile seat, cushion, pillow, and lifestyle to protect your back.

Often people learn to "budget" their back:

After several difficult years, Sam had turned the management of his back pain into a science. He found he could safely pursue certain activities, as long as he didn't try to do too much. If he had a lot of pain, he'd cancel anything that wasn't essential for work so he could go home early and spend the rest of the day lying down.

On a good day, Sam would risk doing more. As long as he knew that he wouldn't be doing too much sitting, he'd try going out to dinner. He'd even take in an occasional movie but would be careful to rest his back earlier in the day. He wasn't going to be stupid, the way he was in the old days, when he frequently pushed himself too hard and paid for it with more pain during the rest of the week.

From past experiences, or from professional advice, many people come to think that they can perform an action only for a given time, lift only a certain weight, or "push" their back only a certain amount each day. Often everything is eventually viewed through the lens of "how it will affect my back."

These concerns all generate anxiety. We fear that we'll pay later for not being careful enough. All of this vigilance causes muscles to tighten and pain to increase. Just how frightened we become depends in large part on what we understand to be the cause of our pain.

Many patients have been told that the disks in their back are like torn "jelly doughnuts" in which the jelly has leaked out. They naturally come to feel that their back is extremely fragile and become frightened of squishing out more "jelly" or rupturing another "doughnut." Others have been told that their spines are "chronically unstable," "arthritic," or "like that of a seventy-year-old person." Perhaps you've heard that your spine is out of alignment or your vertebrae are rubbing against each other. Often it is explained that we have a curvature, short leg, flat feet, or other congenital "malformation," and "it was only a matter of time" before our symptoms would appear. Some patients learn that they are suffering from "degenerative disk disease" which calls up images of our spine deteriorating more and more. All of these diagnoses, quite understandably, make us feel that we are fragile, crippled, and continually in danger of further injury.

Since back pain is so common, these fears are further augmented by all the stories that we hear about other people with "bad backs." There are tales of disability, failed surgeries, and pain that never goes away. Very often we know of a friend or family member with a similar diagnosis and have seen that person limit their life and suffer from ongoing pain. Is it any wonder that many of us become intimidated?

The notion that our spine is injured leads us to avoid activities that we think will harm us further. If we twist an ankle, we generally stay off it until it is no longer very sore. If we burn or cut a finger, we keep it bandaged until the pain subsides. This approach would be effective for us if chronic back pain were indeed due to injuries that rest would heal. Unfortunately, it is completely counterproductive in dealing with a tension problem.

The pain of a chronic back problem is only one example of the body's "guidance" going awry—it happens frequently. Another is the body's defenses reacting to harmless pollen with a full-blown allergy attack.

Sooner or later most people with chronic back pain stop moving the way they used to. This is often made worse by the advice of health care professionals. You may have been told to always bend your knees when you bend over, never arch your back, avoid lifting, sit in special ergonomic chairs, stop jogging, stay off bicycles, avoid sleeping on your stomach, skip the breast stroke, prop yourself up with pillows before having sex, and avoid any sudden movements.

Interestingly, when we ask patients to list the pursuits that they have curtailed, most lists include things that they previously did to relax. Many people with chronic back pain once enjoyed sports, dancing, long walks, working out, and sex, as well as traveling and going to restaurants, sporting events, and movies. When we give these up, we lose important opportunities for unwinding from stress. If you were once athletic, this can be particularly terrible for you. When most athletes stop working out or participating in sports, they quickly become very tense and unhappy. For almost everyone, avoiding activity leads to a buildup of psychological tension.

Another consequence of believing that our back is damaged involves assuming protective postures, often called *bracing* or *guarding*. When we feel pain and believe that we are injured, we naturally try to move in ways to protect the vulnerable part of our body. This often means moving slowly, in a tense, self-conscious manner. Some people come to look a bit like robots or seem to be walking on thin ice as they carefully plan every movement.

Especially for those who have been trained by professionals to be careful, the day is filled with rules. We often learn to favor certain movements and postures over others, becoming quite stiff and unnatural. All of this fearfulness increases emotional and muscular tension, which in turn increases pain.

Another common result of bracing and avoiding everyday exercise is physical *deconditioning*. It is common for people with chronic back pain to rest their backs regularly and avoid even the relatively small amounts of exercise that back muscles automatically receive during the day. Some people also use back supports or corsets, which further inhibit muscle movement. When we limit ourselves in this way, muscles become tighter, shorter, and weaker.

This leaves us vulnerable to minor injuries, in the form of strains and soreness, since even light exercise and normal stretching become a challenge for seriously deconditioned muscles. This brings whole new opportunities for acute back pain, on top of the chronic pain we're already suffering. In addition, it makes us further fear that our backs are fragile, since we lose the confidence that comes from using our backs in the regular way.

It is rather amazing to consider the fact that all these consequences result from one simple mistaken idea. But just as we saw earlier that belief can reduce blood pressure and allow sham treatments to effect a cure, the conviction that our pain is caused by an abnormality can ultimately wreak havoc on our back muscles.

LEARNING TO FEAR

How psychological conditioning causes us to tense our muscles

We have seen how stress, along with believing that our pain is due to a damaged spine, causes all sorts of problems that contribute to the chronic back pain cycle. There are other psychological and physical processes that can exacerbate the problem. One of the more important is known as *classical conditioning.*

Scientists have known for many years that animals (including humans) can be readily conditioned, or trained, to respond to cues that we give to them. Many of these responses involve the activity of the same system that produces the fight-or-flight response. For example, animals can be trained to change their heart rate or digestion in response to a cue, such as a light going on. All that is needed is to initially pair the cue with something that naturally causes the response. The most famous examples of this were Pavlov's experiments in which he trained dogs to salivate to the sound of a bell.

Something similar happens accidentally to most of us with chronic back pain. Life events themselves, rather than an experimenter, pair a variety of cues to pain. We quickly learn conditioned associations between pain and whatever else may be going on at the time we feel it.

For example, if we feel intense pain while sitting one day, the next time we sit down we will begin to have an anxiety or fear response, including an increase in the tightness of our muscles. This will often be accompanied by the thought *I hope that my back doesn't start to hurt like the last time I had to sit.* Since the pain itself will likely be increased by this heightened tension, we will then have a second experience of pain while sitting, which further conditions us to associate sitting with pain.

This same psychological conditioning of muscle tension can occur in connection with virtually any action, such as sitting, standing, walking, driving, bending, or lifting. We naturally figure that it is the physical act that is irritating our injury.

Joseph had struggled with back pain on and off for years. Recently it hadn't bothered him very much. One day, riding home in his car, he passed over one of the many potholes on the street leading up to his house. He felt a bad twinge of pain in his back. He hoped that this wouldn't be the start of another episode.

Later that night, his back started to ache. He feared that going over the pothole had thrown his back out but hoped that he was wrong. By the next morning his back hurt a lot, and he had to struggle to sit at his desk all day at work. That evening he went to his chiropractor, who adjusted him. Over the course of the next few days he felt better. A week later he again hit a bump. He felt another twinge. That night, another backache.

During the next several months, every time Joseph went over a bump in his car, the pain returned. Things like mowing the lawn, food shopping, and vacuuming didn't bother him. He could even work out at the gym without difficulty. Even though he had a good car with a suspension that absorbed bumps pretty well, the bumps always threw his back out.

Joseph tried very hard to avoid going over potholes. He drove slowly, watching the road carefully, and was usually able to steer around the bumps. Still, every once in a while he'd hit one, and his pain would come back.

It is very unlikely that going over small bumps at slow speed in a good car was actually injuring Joseph's back. Because of the sheer power of conditioning, whenever he hit a bump his muscles tensed and his pain returned. He was thus fooled into reacting as though potholes were dangerous.

Naturally, once we develop a fear response to an activity, we try to limit or avoid it. When we return to such an activity, our psychological conditioning makes us tense and often brings on the pain.

A common example of this involves sitting in chairs. Many back pain sufferers have been told that sitting is terrible for their back. As a result, they try to avoid it whenever possible. If they have to sit, they immediately begin to feel tense, anticipating an increase in pain.

Some people continue to have difficulty sitting, even after successfully completing a rehabilitation program in which they learn to lift heavy weights, exercise vigorously, and become limber:

When Allen first began his rehabilitation program, he was afraid to bend from the waist or lift more than a couple of pounds. He relied on others to do most chores and had become quite sedentary.

While he found the program terrifying at first, it eventually had him lifting forty pounds without bending his knees, jogging a couple of miles at a time, and touching his toes. He still felt some pain but was delighted to finally feel strong and healthy.

Despite his renewed confidence, whenever he sat for more than a few minutes, the pain returned. He consequently continued to avoid sitting whenever possible.

It eventually became clear that Allen had developed a conditioned fear of sitting, and no matter how healthy and strong his back felt at other times, he was still afraid of chairs. He eventually had to face this fear by systematically increasing his sitting time, before he could end the pain.

PAVLOV'S BACK?

Developing a phobia of using the back

Much of the early research on psychological conditioning in people was performed to understand *phobias.* These are irrational fears that limit our ability to engage in life.

Some phobias tend to follow a course remarkably similar to that of chronic back pain. The best-known of these, *agoraphobia,* involves being afraid to go out in public. It often begins with a sudden activation of our fight-or-flight reaction, usually in a public place such as the supermarket. The person's heart races, their breath quickens, they sweat profusely, and they feel dizzy or faint. These symptoms together are called a *panic attack.*

These attacks may begin as mild or moderate anxiety. At a certain point the person becomes concerned about the physical manifestations of the anxiety (the fight-or-flight reaction) and may fear that they are having a heart attack or might faint. These frightened thoughts intensify the physical symptoms, which in turn worsens the anxiety. The person rapidly becomes caught in an escalating cycle of physiological arousal and fear, which usually leads to a ride to the emergency room or running out of the place where all of this is happening.

When they return to the place where they had the episode, they typically feel anxious again—a response conditioned by their last experience. This can begin another cycle, which more deeply ingrains the fear.

The process by which people with chronic back pain become afraid of a host of activities is very similar. Instead of fearing the racing heart and breathlessness of agoraphobia, chronic back pain sufferers fear increases in pain. In both problems, people share the mistaken belief that something dangerous is happening when their symptoms appear.

Another similarity between agoraphobia and chronic back pain involves the response to normal levels of discomfort. Once a person has suffered from intense cycles of anxiety and physiological arousal, he or she becomes especially sensitive and reactive to normal anxiety. Thus an agoraphobic person may launch into a vicious cycle of fear and autonomic arousal in response to mild, temporary anxiety, because they fear that it will grow into another intense anxiety attack. This then becomes a self-fulfilling prophecy.

Similarly, most people with chronic back pain become fearful of any pain or soreness in their backs. When pain arises, they fear that it may turn into a serious back pain episode and perhaps cause them to become disabled. They can become quite disturbed by levels of back pain that normal people accept as a common "backache." As a result, ordinary muscle soreness or transient tension can easily develop into serious back pain episodes.

FROM BAD TO WORSE

Frustration, anger, and depression

You have probably consulted with many health care professionals in search of relief from your pain. Most of the people we see have gone through many cycles of hope and disappointment as successive treatments show promise and then fail. Sooner or later most become frustrated, angry, and depressed. These emotions can become like a pattern of bad weather that affects every part of your life. Depending on the intensity of your pain, and the degree to which it interferes with your work and recreation, these feelings can become quite extreme. Many people describe their episodes of chronic back pain as the worst time they've ever had. They become irritable with loved ones, angry with medical providers, and, eventually, despondent.

The anger that chronic back pain brings up can be quite intense. It is easy to become enraged at this injustice.

For some people, the pain itself is so intense and unremitting that it becomes the focus of their emotional distress. They describe feeling drained and depleted by the pain, reluctant to face each new day, oppressed by time itself. Thoughts of reducing the pain in any way possible dominate each waking moment. As the pain persists, many people become desperate to avoid being crippled or in pain for the rest of their life. It is not unusual to become suicidal under these circumstances, thinking that death would finally bring freedom from the pain.

The focus of frustration, anger, and depression varies from person to person:

Ann was a mother with a four-year-old son. She was trained as a computer professional but decided to stay at home to care for her little boy.

One day, while working out, Ann felt a sharp pain in her back. She figured that she had probably pulled a muscle. When the pain didn't go away after a couple of weeks, she saw her doctor. He suggested that she be careful until the pain subsided. Unfortunately, the pain didn't subside. Ann then began a long medical ordeal involving a neurologist, orthopedist, chiropractor, and several physical therapists.

She soon felt that she could barely care for her son and needed her husband's help to make the beds, vacuum the rugs, and do the laundry. She became frustrated and angry and found herself yelling at the boy every time he made a mess. Her sex life fell apart as tensions in the marriage grew. She became increasingly depressed and sometimes just wanted to die. Only her love for her son and husband kept her going.

Your particular experience may be different, but you probably have some things in common with Ann and other chronic back pain sufferers. Most often people are more concerned about being disabled or missing out on life than about the pain itself. For those people who have lost their jobs because of chronic back pain, feelings of inadequacy, disappointment, and frustration usually center around being unemployed and feeling unproductive. For people who have given up athletic and recreational pursuits, missing these can be central.

Most chronic back pain sufferers find that their family relationships and friendships suffer because of their condition and often become very upset about this. Our bad moods push others away, and other people may become tired of taking care of us. We frequently feel that we cannot safely enjoy sex, and this too interferes with relationships. Like Ann, most parents with chronic back pain feel terrible remorse about not being the kind of parent they would like to be, either because they are irritable or because they can't take care of their children adequately and play with them the way they want to.

Our everyday experience shows us that there is a close relationship among frustration, anger, and tightening of muscles. Imagine for a moment that you are very angry. Now act this out with your body. You will probably notice tension, perhaps centered in the shoulders, neck, and upper back. As the "fight" component of the fight-or-flight response, frustration and anger bring with them distinctive patterns of muscle tension that worsen our pain.

HOW CHRONIC BACK PAIN CAUSES DEPRESSION

It will probably come as no surprise to you that research shows depression to be very common in people with chronic back pain. Depending on how it is defined, somewhere between 50 percent and 90 percent of people with chronic back pain also suffer from some degree of depression. People with chronic back pain are *three to four times* more likely to suffer from *serious* depression than the general population.

There are several ways of understanding how this depression develops. While depression has many roots, research shows that feelings of frustration and anger can turn to depression, if we have no outlet for acknowledging or expressing them. This observation goes all the way back to Freud. These feelings are turned against the self, resulting in the self-criticism and gloomy outlook characteristic of depression.

It is not hard to see how this process might unfold in someone suffering from chronic back pain. Many people feel that there is no place to direct angry feelings, especially if they are dependent on, and protective of, loved ones and need their health care providers to help them. This can lead to depression, which reduces the hope and motivation necessary to work at getting better.

Another source of depression, called *learned helplessness,* involves the tendency to give up after repeated failures. After countless unsuccessful treatments, it is easy to conclude that nothing will help. Learned helplessness can make us quite reluctant to try a new solution to our problems or persist in the face of difficulties.

The concept of learned helplessness is based on animal studies. Dogs were placed in a cage, to which an electric shock was applied. The dogs whimpered, howled, and tried to escape at first, but they eventually gave up and lay on the floor. They

showed physiological stress responses that we associate with depression, lost interest in food, and no longer played. The next day the dogs were placed in a cage that was electrified on only one side, so that they could easily escape the shock. Unlike normal dogs, the "depressed" animals made no effort to escape. Even when they occasionally wandered over, they didn't learn from their experience. The dogs had learned to be helpless, and this looked a lot like human depression.

You may have noticed that when you feel depressed, you are critical of yourself and pessimistic about the future. Often these thoughts are not logical, but they are very powerful. You may think it is your fault that you engaged in the activity you believed caused your pain, or you may blame yourself for not getting good enough medical attention. Perhaps you've decided that your pain is punishment for some failure. The plain truth is, nobody knows why some people develop chronic back pain while others suffer from other stress-related maladies. Later on we will help you deal with the self-critical thoughts that you may be having.

This brings to a close our overview of the chronic back pain cycle illustrated in figure 3. We have seen that most people suffering from chronic back pain come to believe that something in their spine is defective. We have described the cycles that then become established, in which pain causes anxiety, fear, or aggravation, which in turn causes increased muscle tightness, followed by intensified pain and emotional upset. We have also seen how easily we can become conditioned to feel fear, tension, and pain in response to a variety of activities or situations and how this leads us to restrict our movements. This restriction leads to more fear, lost opportunities to relax, and physical deconditioning.

Even if these ideas make complete sense to you, you may not be able to abandon your worries until you've seen them work in your own mind and body. The next section of the book, "Relieving Chronic Back Pain," will help you do that. Curing chronic back pain requires interrupting the cycle. You have already begun that process by questioning your assumptions about what has caused your pain.

PART 2

RELIEVING CHRONIC BACK PAIN

CHAPTER

7

BELIEF AND THE BODY

THIS CHAPTER EXPLAINS:

- **How to evaluate your own ideas about which activities are damaging to your back**
- **How to observe the connections among emotion, muscle tension, and pain in your own body**
- **Why "let the pain be your guide" is a good rule of thumb for dealing with many acute injuries but is counterproductive for handling chronic back pain**
- **How recent research shows how caution and rest actually *create* chronic back pain**

At this point we are assuming that you have had a competent medical evaluation (as described in chapter 4) and that you are not one of the rare individuals suffering from one of the unusual medical disorders that can cause back pain and requires special treatment. If all this is true, you are ready to take the next steps toward getting well.

RECOVERING FROM CHRONIC BACK PAIN

Beginning to undo your own cycle of chronic back pain

To recover from chronic back pain, it is important to address each part of the pain cycle. Having (hopefully) understood the "general" dynamics of chronic back pain, you are now ready to turn your attention to the specific chain of events that cause and maintain *your* back pain, as well as to the steps necessary to work your way out of it. These steps will be somewhat different for every reader, but they essentially entail the following:

- **Challenging *your* personal beliefs about what causes your pain**
- **Learning to resume full physical activity**
- **Working with your particular negative thoughts and emotions**
- **Cultivating the most effective ways of dealing with your ongoing stress and important relationships**

EXAMINING PERSONAL BELIEFS

Analyzing the components of your own case

In chapter 2 we asked you to fill out the "Beliefs About Pain" questionnaire. Take a few moments now to look at it again.

Has your understanding of your pain changed since filling it out, or do you feel that "muscle tension may be the problem for others, but my pain is due to my bad ______" (disk, posture, facet joint, alignment, or other diagnosis)? Perhaps you suspect that the doctors have "missed something." These thoughts are common for people during the beginning stages of the Back Sense program. Most people with chronic back pain have been through many failed treatments. It is only natural to be extremely skeptical about yet another new idea.

We do not expect you to give up concerns about your back being damaged right away, and it is not necessary for success with the program. The process of disrupting the pain cycle is a gradual one, and notions about the cause of pain shift little by little, as you begin to experience moments in which your pain does not follow the patterns you had expected. All that is necessary at this point is to

- **believe that tight muscles *may* at least be a part of your pain.**
- **consider the possibility that the activities you believe aggravate your condition may not actually cause any permanent damage to your back.**

We will address these one at a time.

COULD MUSCLE TENSION BE A CAUSE OF YOUR BACK PAIN?

Seeing the role of tight muscles for yourself

Working successfully with your own beliefs involves personal experimentation. You'll need to make your own observations about how your pain responds to different situations. A good place to begin is by examining the relationships among pain level, mood, and muscle tension in your body.

Many people find it helps them to keep a written record of their pain levels for a week or two in order to notice connections between emotions and pain. The "Tracking Your Pain and Emotions" chart will help you do this. It's very simple to use. Make several photocopies of the chart. Throughout each day, note the situation you're in, your emotions at the time, and your pain on a scale from 0 to 10, where 0 is no pain and 10 is extreme pain.

TRACKING YOUR PAIN AND EMOTIONS

Date: ______________________________

TIME	SITUATION	PAIN LEVEL (CIRCLE)	EMOTIONS
7:00 A.M.		0 1 2 3 4 5 6 7 8 9 10	
8:00 A.M.		0 1 2 3 4 5 6 7 8 9 10	
9:00 A.M.		0 1 2 3 4 5 6 7 8 9 10	
10:00 A.M.		0 1 2 3 4 5 6 7 8 9 10	
11:00 A.M.		0 1 2 3 4 5 6 7 8 9 10	
12:00 P.M.		0 1 2 3 4 5 6 7 8 9 10	
1:00 P.M.		0 1 2 3 4 5 6 7 8 9 10	
2:00 P.M.		0 1 2 3 4 5 6 7 8 9 10	
3:00 P.M.		0 1 2 3 4 5 6 7 8 9 10	
4:00 P.M.		0 1 2 3 4 5 6 7 8 9 10	
5:00 P.M.		0 1 2 3 4 5 6 7 8 9 10	
6:00 P.M.		0 1 2 3 4 5 6 7 8 9 10	
7:00 P.M.		0 1 2 3 4 5 6 7 8 9 10	
8:00 P.M.		0 1 2 3 4 5 6 7 8 9 10	
9:00 P.M.		0 1 2 3 4 5 6 7 8 9 10	
10:00 P.M.		0 1 2 3 4 5 6 7 8 9 10	
11:00 P.M.		0 1 2 3 4 5 6 7 8 9 10	

Try observing whether your pain level seems to increase when you are emotionally tense or upset. Has your pain felt worse when something discouraging happened with your back? Is it worse when you have an argument? Is it worse when things go wrong in your day?

When Roger first developed back pain, he was sure that it was because of lifting heavy boxes during his move to a new apartment. It was still bothering him a year later, even though he had been careful to avoid reinjuring himself.

When asked to keep track of his pain levels, Roger noticed that the pain was often worst early in the work week. He had thought that this was because of the lifting that he had to do in his job. When questioned, however, he began to realize that his pain was most serious when he was aggravated at work and tended to feel better over the weekend.

Notice if your pain level decreases at all during more relaxing moments in your daily life. Does it diminish after a massage, hot bath, sauna, or other relaxing activity? Does it decrease when you have fewer responsibilities? Is your pain lessened when you drink alcohol or take "muscle relaxants"?

Russ was suffering with chronic back pain. A friend recommended a masseuse. While the first massage was frightening because of how hard the masseuse pressed, Russ soon learned that it brought relief. It didn't take long to discover that a stiff drink helped, too. Unfortunately, the effects of the massage wore off in a few hours, and drinking all day to reduce the pain wasn't an entirely practical solution.

If, like most chronic back pain sufferers, you have always thought your pain was due to a damaged spine, you may not have noticed these sorts of relationships between life situations and pain before. Try observing your experience through this new lens. Fill in copies of the "Tracking Your Pain and Emotions" chart over the next week. See whether any patterns emerge that are consistent with the idea that emotional distress contributes to your pain.

One particular emotional experience is almost guaranteed to make back pain better or worse—the diagnosis you get from your doctor. You may recall from Dr. Siegel's story how unhappy he was after being told that he had a herniated disk and how this sparked a serious downhill slide. Many of our patients have similar experiences, in which their pain increases after receiving a distressing diagnosis.

Evelyn had dealt with moderate back pain for many years. She had a high-powered job and figured that her back hurt because she never had time to get enough exercise or rest. Around the time of her fiftieth birthday, the pain became more intense and more persistent. Her doctor sent her to an orthopedist. He ordered an MRI and told her that three of the disks in her lower back had degenerated. After hearing this, Evelyn's pain became worse and she grew very depressed about her situation.

On the other hand, an upbeat medical assessment can bring considerable relief. This turns out to be a key factor in the apparent success of many treatments that don't address stress directly. Patients are given hopeful diagnoses and are reassured that their doctor can cure them. They then start to relax and consequently feel better.

Martha had been very dejected about her back pain for a year. She had given up most of what she enjoyed and spent a lot of her time going to doctors and trying different treatments, but she was still in agony much of the time. She missed many days at work and was afraid that her boss wouldn't put up with her much longer.

Martha now dates the beginning of her recovery to a visit with a doctor specializing in rehabilitation. The physician examined her, took a look at her MRI, and concluded that her structural "problems" were minor and weren't causing her pain. He told her that he could help her to get back into shape and that her pain would probably lessen as a result.

The next week, even before beginning rehabilitation, Martha began to feel better. Just the thought that she might not *be crippled helped her to relax and reduced her pain.*

Has your back "reacted" to hopeful, or discouraging, news? While not true for everyone, this is one way that many people first see for themselves that emotional events have a direct impact on our experience of pain.

HAZARDOUS CAUTION

Why it is better for most people to exercise despite pain

Take a moment, again, to review your "Beliefs About Pain" questionnaire. If you are like most chronic back pain sufferers, you've worked hard to figure out exactly which activities seem to make your back better or worse. We can become like zealous scientists, tracking whether our pain gets worse after we sit too long, stand too long, lie down too long, lift too much, twist too much, or use the wrong mattress, chair, or car seat. You may have "discovered" these relationships and become convinced that certain activities make your pain worse. Naturally, you'd be inclined to try to avoid those activities.

We automatically assume that the actions that seem to increase our pain are worsening our condition. Some people worry that they are making their bulging disks protrude more or damaging other disks. Others believe that they are irritating or damaging nerves through activity and will have to pay for it later with hours or days of pain and increased disability. Sometimes people fear that they are injuring an already damaged muscle, ligament, or tendon when their pain increases.

Jerry found that sitting for any significant period of time worsened his pain. He had been given a diagnosis of a herniated disk in his lower back and had been told that sitting placed tremendous pressure on the spine.

Jerry had been told by his doctor that disks are like jelly doughnuts, and once they rupture, pressure forces the softer inner "jelly" against nerve roots. Whenever he sat, he imagined this process and thought that he might wind up completely crippled.

Pain appears to alert us to illness or injury and prompts us to take steps to protect ourselves. Understanding this leads us to believe that we should "let pain be our guide" and stop any activities that appear to cause discomfort. If our chronic back pain were really caused by an unhealed injury, that would be true, but it is a very poor strategy for dealing with chronic back pain. Because chronic pain is really due to muscle tension and disuse, exercise is beneficial. The fact that it hurts does not mean you are damaging yourself. We cannot emphasize this point enough. Avoiding activity only adds to our problems.

We saw in chapter 6 how psychological conditioning can cause us to experience pain in association with virtually any endeavor. Once we feel increased pain in connection with an activity, we associate that activity with pain and (often without even being aware of it) become fearful whenever we engage in it again. This in turn intensifies our pain. When psychological conditioning is the cause, listening to pain only deepens our conditioned fear.

Many scientific studies, from all over the world, show that becoming fearful of activity can cause acute back pain to become chronic. In fact, research shows that it is *usually* the fear of pain, rather than its intensity, that causes people to become disabled.

Our experience supports this idea. Many back pain sufferers are astounded to learn that others with the exact same condition fear completely opposite things. Some complain about sitting, others standing. Some people are convinced that doing a specific exercise is a problem, while others blame not doing it.

After searching for almost a year, Richard discovered just the bed he needed to keep his back pain tolerable—a top-of-the-line extra-firm mattress. It had been an expensive quest, because he first bought, and then gave away, three other beds. With this arrangement, he could finally sleep through the night on occasion. Of course, traveling was an ordeal, because hotels hadn't seen fit to make the same investment in his back comfort.

To begin to get better, it is important to examine all of the activities that you associate with pain and ask yourself whether your assumptions about them causing damage hold up. The back is made up of bones, disks, ligaments, tendons, and muscles. Muscles, tendons, and ligaments are made of durable fibers, and the rest is made of either bone or gristle. Does it really make sense that these materials would be badly damaged by everyday movement?

Why is one person "damaged" by sitting while another's problems are made worse by lying down? Just about all of our patients eventually discover mistaken logic in their reasoning about the effect of activity on their backs. It is not that they are irrational people, it is just that they haven't had any other way to understand their pain, and our minds are always searching for explanations to make sense of our experience.

YOUR BACK IS NOT A FRAGILE FLOWER

Realizing your back is strong

To support your progress, begin thinking of your back as strong and stable. It actually is.

John had a demanding job and a busy family life. One day at work he bent over to pick up a box and felt a pop in his back, followed by intense pain. Ten months later he was barely capable of dragging himself to the job. He endured medication, injections, massage, physical therapy, and chiropractic adjustments. On doctors' advice he avoided sitting for long periods, skipped heavy lifting, and always bent his knees. Nothing helped.

In dire straits, he went to a rehabilitation center that was supposed to be different. He had heard that one before. He was brought into an exercise room where an elderly woman was lifting plastic milk crates filled with heavy weights. She was panting and sweating, moving them on and off industrial shelving. He couldn't believe his eyes. She wasn't bending her knees or practicing any of the "safe" lifting he had been taught. Was this some sort of weird science experiment gone awry?

In a state of near alarm, John went over to talk with the woman. He was shocked to learn that she had a long history of pain and disability. She said that she was beginning to live a normal life for the first time in years.

Programs like the one John visited have been shown to reduce pain significantly. The field of rehabilitation medicine is increasingly embracing them. It is therefore very important to start thinking of exercise as being beneficial for pain rather than dangerous.

We know that most of you, like John, will have trouble accepting this at first. Remember the research showing that people in nonindustrialized societies experience far less chronic back pain despite doing far more strenuous physical labor.

Many studies have compared the clinical course of patients with acute back pain who rest extensively with that of patients who keep up normal activities despite distress.

In one study, city workers who came to a clinic with acute back pain were given differing treatments. Some were told to rest in bed for two days, some were given back exercises, and the third group was told to go about their normal activities. The normal activity group had the shortest-lasting pain and the best work attendance records.

Many other studies have had similar results. Research has also demonstrated the benefits of intense exercise for people with chronic back pain. Here are examples:

A very large study compared vigorous exercise with rest and medication for people disabled by back pain. They found that the people who exercised despite their pain *returned to work more quickly than those receiving conventional treatments.*

A colleague of ours did an interesting study that looked at people's notions about which movements or activities would cause them pain and what they could actually accomplish through strength and flexibility training. In the course of an aggressive exercise program, patients were able to significantly improve their physical capacity without any significant increase in pain. This happened despite their believing *that the exercises would significantly increase their pain.*

Finally, you should know that recent research proves that the instructions on careful lifting, ergonomic chairs, and proper posture that you may have been taught (possibly in so-called back school) have been shown to be ineffective in both preventing and curing back pain:

> *A major study, published in the* New England Journal of Medicine, *involved four thousand postal workers. Half of them received repeated professional training in back safety, correct lifting, and posture; the other half were given no instruction. Over more than five years, there were no differences between the two groups in either incidence of back pain or speed of recovery from episodes.*

Many other studies of back school programs have reached the same conclusion. Taken together with research on the effects of rest versus exercise, being careful actually appears to be harmful.

In determining how aggressively to pursue resuming activity, it is of course sensible to consider your current level of strength and flexibility so as to not overdo it. At the same time, even if you've chosen the perfect starting point, you may well experience increased pain. Remember, though, that the pain is harmless.

It is important to discover this through your own experience. One of the first things to consider in this regard is the variability of your pain. Many people find that there are some days in which a given activity is associated with considerable pain, but other days in which the same activity does not seem to cause much increase in pain at all. If you fill out the "Tracking Your Pain and Emotions" chart for a few weeks, you'll probably notice this. This strongly suggests that the activity per se is not damaging the back, but that other factors account for the coming and going of the pain.

For most people, the best way to evaluate this is to experiment with abandoned activities that they have associated with pain in the past. This can require a good deal of bravery at first. You will eventually see that carrying out such activity actually only causes discomfort—however formidable—from using weakened muscles and fears of exceeding your supposed limits. This is the focus of the next chapter.

CHAPTER 8

RESTORING YOUR LIFE

THIS CHAPTER EXPLAINS:

- Why waiting for your pain to go away before resuming activity doesn't work
- How to undertake a safe and effective rehabilitation program
- How to develop attitudes that enhance the pace of your return to wellness

RESUMING ACTIVITY

Steps toward recapturing functioning

You are probably beginning to see that unrestricted movement should pose little danger to your back. We hope that you feel ready enough to take the next steps. If you have become limited in your activities, shifting your goal from reducing pain to increasing movement is warranted.

Most of us with chronic back pain, quite naturally, focus our efforts on alleviating the pain. This reaction is "hardwired" in people—we all want relief. Unfortunately, like many of our other natural reactions and assumptions regarding chronic back pain, this attitude keeps us stuck in the syndrome. It does so in two major ways.

First, *as long as you are trying to get rid of pain, you stay preoccupied with it.* Constant monitoring of our pain level keeps the mind full of worried thoughts about how one activity or another is going to affect it, and these anxious thoughts result in increased tension.

Second, *by trying to avoid pain, you avoid the activities that you associate with it.* This results in an increasing fear of "risky" movements so that we become anxious whenever engaging in them. Avoiding activity also leads to a loss of muscle condition, which makes us vulnerable to all sorts of acute injuries. Consider what happened to Andrea:

> *Andrea suffered from chronic back pain with sciatica for years. She regularly went to the chiropractor, who adjusted her spine and gave her ultrasound and electrical stimulation treatments. These made her feel better temporarily, but the pain always came back. Andrea was depressed—constantly preoccupied with how much she was hurting, and struggling to decide whether the chiropractic treatments were actually helping.*
>
> *While Andrea was able to work, she had stopped going to movies (too much sitting), taking walks, and gardening (too much bending). She was waiting for chiropractic treatment to make the pain go away before returning to these beloved pursuits. Like most health care providers, Andrea's chiropractor was completely focused on finding a way to reduce her pain. He didn't want to risk "making things worse" by pushing her before her back was "healed."*
>
> *Unfortunately, time was passing, but her back pain was undiminished.*

While well intentioned, this sort of attempt to alleviate pain can keep you trapped. We are not suggesting that you need to live with the pain forever. Instead, we are saying that at this stage in the program it is most important to devote yourself to reclaiming lost activities. Leading a full and interesting life is the best way to reduce your problematic focus on pain. Returning to normal activity will also bring your muscles back to natural levels of strength and flexibility and allow you once again to participate in stress-reducing, life-enhancing pursuits. The key point is that as you start to live normally and feel less emotional distress, the pain will begin to go away *by itself.*

The cycle of chronic back pain is then replaced by a new sequence of increased movement, growing confidence, reduced tension, and reduced pain. In this new recovery cycle, illustrated in figure 4, your self-assurance will grow as tension and pain gradually diminish. You will become capable of taking on more and more until you no longer think of yourself as someone with a bad back at all.

WHERE DO I BEGIN?

A map for charting your course

Your first increases in exertion are usually the hardest, because they tend to be the most intimidating. The "Lost Activities" chart will help you assess the ways in which chronic back pain has limited your life. You can then use this information to choose the best way to begin.

Use the chart to list all of the activities that you used to engage in, however long ago, that you have given up or limited because of back pain. We have suggested several categories. The particular endeavors you have curtailed may fall into these areas or may fit into the "other" category.

Once you complete the list, rate your feeling about each one before you developed back pain. Was it pleasant, unpleasant, or neutral? Check the appropriate box.

Next rate how difficult you imagine it would be to resume each pursuit. Do you think it would be easy, moderate, or difficult? Again, check the appropriate box.

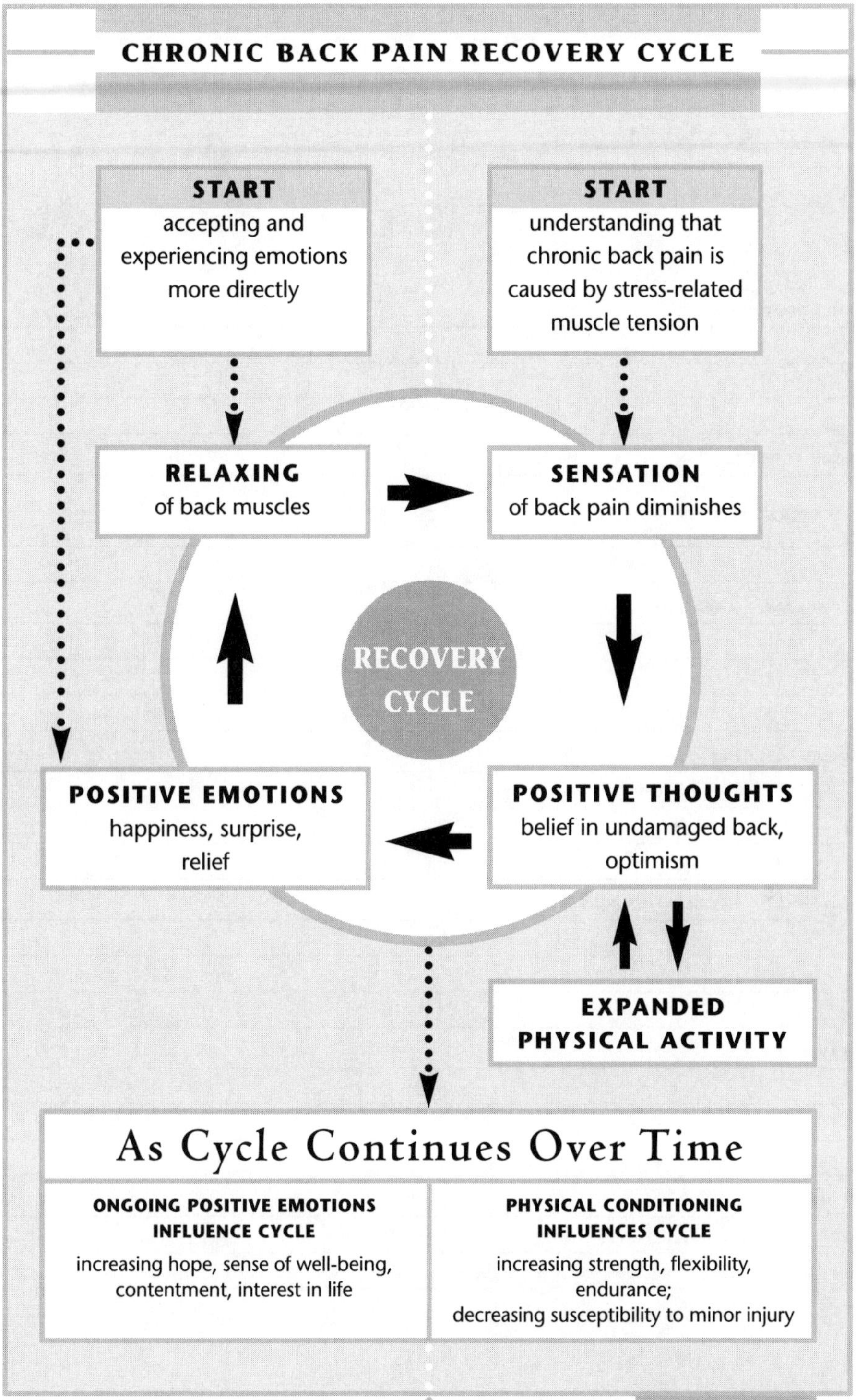
CHRONIC BACK PAIN RECOVERY CYCLE
START
accepting and experiencing emotions more directly
START
understanding that chronic back pain is caused by stress-related muscle tension
RELAXING
of back muscles
SENSATION
of back pain diminishes
RECOVERY CYCLE
POSITIVE EMOTIONS
happiness, surprise, relief
POSITIVE THOUGHTS
belief in undamaged back, optimism
EXPANDED PHYSICAL ACTIVITY
As Cycle Continues Over Time
ONGOING POSITIVE EMOTIONS INFLUENCE CYCLE
increasing hope, sense of well-being, contentment, interest in life
PHYSICAL CONDITIONING INFLUENCES CYCLE
increasing strength, flexibility, endurance;
decreasing susceptibility to minor injury

Figure 4

LOST ACTIVITIES

CATEGORY	SPECIFIC ACTIVITY	PLEASANT	NEUTRAL	UNPLEASANT		EASY	MODERATE	DIFFICULT
DAILY ROUTINES								
WORK ACTIVITIES								
SPORTS AND RECREATION								
SOCIAL ACTIVITIES								
PERSONAL/FAMILY RELATIONSHIPS								
TRAVEL								
OTHER								

Look now at your completed "Lost Activities" chart. Circle the ones that you rated both pleasant and easy. Which of these could you engage in three or more times per week if you weren't limited by your pain? Which one do you feel would be most rewarding or relaxing to reclaim? We have found that this is the best place to begin.

Depending on your particular situation, you might choose a relatively light activity such as walking, bicycle riding, or cooking. If you are already somewhat active, you might identify a more strenuous pursuit such as tennis, basketball, dancing, aerobics, or weight lifting. It all depends on what you used to enjoy doing, how constricted your life has become, and what your schedule permits.

Tom felt his back "go out" one day while working at a printing press. He returned to work but was assigned light duty and now avoids lifting heavy stacks of paper or sitting for long periods. At home he also shuns lifting and sitting. He is most unhappy that he can't even pick up his four-year-old son. The boy cries and pleads when Tom says no. He has largely abandoned recreation, except for things he can do while lying down.

Look at Tom's chart on the next page. You can see that Tom checked "Neighborhood walks" and "Swimming at the YMCA" as pleasant activities that would be relatively easy to resume. He can do either one four times per week. Tom feels that walking would be most relaxing. For him, this is a good place to start.

If you have not engaged in your chosen pursuit recently (within the past month) and have not been physically active in general, you have probably lost much of the strength, flexibility, and endurance that you once had. Gentle actions such as walking can usually be undertaken safely right away, while more vigorous endeavors may require a more gradual reentry. There are several reasons to avoid rushing right back in. First, your heart and lungs may not be used to exercise, and they need to be conditioned gradually. (In chapter 13 you can find guidelines for evaluating your level of fitness and finding the optimal level of exertion with which to begin more intensive exercise.) Second, you can expect that you will experience some normal muscle soreness as you begin to work neglected muscle groups, and there is no reason to create

LOST ACTIVITIES

CATEGORY	SPECIFIC ACTIVITY	PLEASANT	NEUTRAL	UNPLEASANT	EASY	MODERATE	DIFFICULT
DAILY ROUTINES	Doing dishes		✓		✓		
	Food shopping			✓	✓		
	Shoveling snow		✓				✓
	Mowing the lawn		✓			✓	
WORK ACTIVITIES	Lifting paper bales		✓				✓
	Sitting to operate presses	✓					✓
	Cleaning presses			✓			✓
SPORTS AND RECREATION	Swimming at the YMCA	✓			✓		
	Neighborhood walks	✓			✓		
	Tennis	✓					✓
	Bike riding	✓					✓
SOCIAL ACTIVITIES	Movies	✓				✓	
	Restaurants	✓				✓	
	Ball games	✓				✓	
	Parties	✓				✓	
PERSONAL/FAMILY RELATIONSHIPS	Lifting my son	✓					✓
	Roughousing with my son	✓					✓
	Sexual relations	✓					✓
	Visiting my sister	✓				✓	
TRAVEL	Driving for more than 20 minutes		✓			✓	
	Airplane trips	✓					✓
OTHER	Working on my car		✓				✓
	Teaching my son to ride his bike	✓				✓	

unnecessary pain. Finally, starting slowly helps to make fear of movement more manageable. You wouldn't have stopped doing something gratifying in the first place unless you believed it would be harmful to continue.

PERSISTING WITH ACTIVITY

Unlearning avoidance

Most chronic back pain sufferers constantly monitor their pain level to determine what makes it better or worse. They then come to fear those activities and feel pain when they engage in them. When pursuing an activity, there are several guidelines you should follow that will help to eliminate these troublesome responses:

1. Create a regular schedule and stick to it. This should involve repeating the activity in a similar fashion at least three times per week. By regularly repeating the same movements and positions, you will eventually find that the amount of pain fluctuates from day to day while your physical movements remain the same. This will help to weaken the psychologically conditioned association between the activity and the pain, which will in turn lessen your fear.

2. Perform the activity for the same duration and with the same intensity each time. For instance, if your activity is walking, it is important to decide on a distance or time for your walks and an approximate speed. You might decide to walk for fifteen minutes at a normal walking pace or six blocks at a leisurely pace. If you are working out using machines or weights, you would pick a length of time or number of repetitions, along with an amount of resistance or weight to use. Try not to reduce your duration or intensity just because it hurt last time. If you can do your activity consistently, you will gradually come to see that variations in your pain are not due simply to changes in your activity level. This will further weaken the association between activity and pain.

3. Try not to stop the activity early because of discomfort. Stop at your goal rather than when the pain gets too intense. Discontinuing an activity prematurely, or continuing past your goal until you experience serious pain, trains you to escape and avoid it. As you will see later, this can create real problems for your program.

4. Try to move normally when doing the activity. As we said, one of our instinctive responses to pain is to "brace" the body to protect the sore area. Bracing contributes to overall tightness of muscles and therefore to pain. To counteract this, notice any bracing and try to move like a normal person. It also helps to maintain regular breathing, since people often hold their breath when fearful.

5. Visualize doing the activity in the normal way. By *imagining* our body moving as we wish, we can actually facilitate the movement. Professional athletes often use this technique: Take some quiet time and picture yourself performing the movements and positions you have chosen to recapture. Imagine yourself doing them confidently. Remember how good it used to feel. Visualize the muscles loosening and blood flowing to the area that hurts.

When muscles have been tight for a long time, or have gone into spasm, certain postures and movements are acutely painful. This can make it exceptionally difficult to move. Sometimes we feel intense "nerve pain," and it may be torture to bend beyond a certain point or flex a particular muscle.

It is important to know that this type of pain is almost always quite harmless. But if you encounter it, you may not feel *able* to move right. There is no need to force yourself into intolerable pain. Instead, try to move as normally as you can without pushing past this point. You will eventually find yourself able to move properly again. If you are very stiff, refer to chapter 13 for gentle stretching exercises that will help to increase your range of motion.

You can keep a written record of your planned activity with the following chart (make several copies first):

ACTIVITY PLAN

ACTIVITY: ______________________________

FREQUENCY: ______________________________

(How often you will do it—times per week)

DURATION: ______________________________

(How long you will do it—distance, time, or number of repetitions)

INTENSITY: ______________________________

(How hard it will be—speed, weight, or resistance)

Here is what Tom's first activity plan looked like:

ACTIVITY PLAN

ACTIVITY: Walking in neighborhood

FREQUENCY: Four times/week: Monday, Wednesday, Friday, and Sunday

(How often you will do it—times per week)

DURATION: 20 minutes/day

(How long you will do it—distance, time, or number of repetitions)

INTENSITY: Leisurely pace

(How hard it will be—speed, weight, or resistance)

While you engage in your chosen pursuit, observe your thoughts and emotional reactions. Do doubts and worries arise? Do you have concerns that you are damaging yourself or setting yourself up for more pain? Do you worry that we are giving you unsound advice? These sorts of thoughts are practically a given. They will almost certainly change as you stick with the schedule. Most people find that their anxious thoughts increase when the pain increases and diminish when the pain diminishes.

After pursuing this for a few weeks, most people will notice at least one instance in which the activity does *not* seem to make their pain worse. If the movements were actually damaging, they would cause pain every time they were performed, without exception. Therefore it is crucially important to notice when this does *not* happen. This very personal discovery—that a previously feared movement is not, in fact, causing harm—can be a giant confidence builder.

Tom had very mixed feelings about beginning his walking program. The idea that stress was part of his problem made sense, but pushing himself to do things in the past had always backfired, causing more pain later. Despite his doubts, he was fed up with being disabled. He was ready to try something new.

The first few times he took his twenty-minute walk, things didn't go well at all. His back hurt even before beginning and got tighter and tighter as he went on. Sometimes his sciatica became really intense, and he feared that he wouldn't be able to continue. He was beginning to think that this new program was a mistake. It took significant courage to continue.

After the first week, Tom was pretty sure that his back and leg had gotten worse. He needed a good deal of encouragement to resume walking the second week. Again the pain continued, but he noticed that it seemed to be leveling off. This was a relief, since it suggested that at least the walks weren't causing any serious damage.

Finally, during the third week, Tom had an experience where his back actually felt better after walking. This was a happy surprise indeed. Even when the pain returned the next day, he still felt optimistic.

He continued with the plan. Some days his back hurt more, some days a little less. Sometimes his sciatica was more intense, other days it seemed to fade. It became clear that his pain level wasn't closely tied to his walking regimen at all. He actually started looking forward to the walks and began to have the first positive feelings about using his body that he had experienced since his back went out.

We have found that Tom's pattern is not unusual at all. People often experience an initial increase in pain when they resume doing things they used to do. If they pursue it regularly, however, the pain returns to normal or diminishes, usually within a few weeks.

It is vital to remind yourself over and over that you are not trying to get the pain to go away at this point. If we wait for the pain to go away before returning to life, we may wait a lifetime. On the other hand, if we learn through experience that increasing activity does not in itself permanently increase our pain, then we can happily resume our lives.

FIXING A PHOBIA

How to unlearn fear of movement

Here's another way to think about what we are trying to accomplish. We have discussed the similarities between chronic back pain and phobias. Anxiety plays a major role in both of these difficulties. While there are many treatments for anxiety, some of the most effective ones are very similar to the process we have been describing. They use a well-proven psychological principle called *exposure treatment.* The core of this procedure is to expose a person to the feared object or situation, then help that person to resist fleeing in response to the initially uncomfortable physical sensations or worried thoughts that occur. It involves learning to gradually face our fears until our anxiety subsides by itself. Once dreaded actions are repeated until they feel like "no big deal."

Hundreds of research studies confirm that this technique effectively cures a variety of anxiety problems.

Here's an example of how exposure treatment works: Some people develop an overwhelming fear of snakes. They actually refuse to go anyplace where there is even a remote chance of meeting up with one. Treatment starts by bringing the person into a room with a snake locked in a cage several yards away. The person stays there until he or she calms down and no longer feels like running out. Next the snake, in its cage, is moved a few feet closer. The person becomes frightened again but is encouraged to stay there until the fear subsides. This process is repeated, each time moving the snake a little closer. Eventually the cage is opened. If a person sticks with the program to the point of actually handling the snake, the phobia usually disappears.

During this kind of treatment two important things happen. First, the person learns that it is possible to bear the discomfort of an intense fight-or-flight reaction. Second, through repeated experiences in which nothing disastrous happens, the problematic association between the feared object or situation and the anxiety symptoms gradually weakens.

In the Back Sense program we use the same principles to overcome fears of injuring our back. First, by repeating an activity on a regular schedule, you learn that you can tolerate discomfort, and that performing the activity causes no lasting damage. Second, you gradually break the association between the activity and pain, so you can eventually pursue the activity with greatly diminished concern. Your thoughts, bodily reactions, and behaviors simultaneously begin to change for the better.

REWARDING SUCCESS

How to turn psychological conditioning to your own advantage

The psychological conditioning produced by reward and punishment also exerts a powerful effect on pain cycles. If a certain action or behavior is followed by a pleasurable consequence (rewarded), we are more likely to repeat that action. If, on the other hand, a behavior is followed by an unpleasant consequence (punished), we are less prone to repeat it.

With phobias and other anxiety problems, we are inadvertently rewarded each time we withdraw from a feared object or situation. If we become anxious about snakes when walking in a park and get relief when we return to the road, that relief in effect rewards our departure and makes us more likely to flee the park next time. Similarly, in treating chronic back pain, if you quit an activity in response to pain and experience relief, quitting is rewarded, and you become more prone to quit or avoid that activity again.

This pattern of escape and avoidance is known to be one of the toughest behavior patterns to change without a structured program. Left to our own devices, we have a compelling inclination to simply continue the avoidance. Because of this, we never get to have the experience of sticking with a difficult situation long enough to see our fear subside on its own.

The Back Sense program tackles this problem by systematically supporting your persistence in feared pursuits until you are rewarded by fading anxiety and diminished pain. This makes it much easier to remain with an activity the next time you feel uncomfortable. Then a positive momentum begins to build on itself. When Tom discovered in the third week that his pain occasionally lessened after walking, it became easier for him to continue.

The principle of reward can be mobilized to your advantage by keeping a log of your progress in regaining activities. It can be very heartening to see yourself recovering, and this reinforces your efforts. The "Tracking Your Progress" chart is a good way to do that. (Photocopy the chart first.) It will help you to see how long you've continued an activity and to track increases in duration and intensity. You can also use it to observe how your emotional reactions to the pain change over time.

TRACKING YOUR PROGRESS

Activity: ______________________________

Planned Frequency: ______________________________

(How often you plan to do it—times per week)

DATE	**DURATION** *(how long you did it—distance, time, or number of repetitions)*	**INTENSITY** *(how hard it was—speed, weight, or resistance)*	**EMOTIONAL REACTIONS**

Here is what Tom's chart looked like when he began his walking program:

TRACKING YOUR PROGRESS

Activity: Walking in Neighborhood

Planned Frequency: Four times per week: Monday, Wednesday, Friday, and Sunday

(How often you plan to do it—times per week)

DATE	DURATION *(how long you did it—distance, time, or number of repetitions)*	INTENSITY *(how hard it was—speed, weight, or resistance)*	EMOTIONAL REACTIONS
4/3/00	20 minutes	Leisurely	Scared, hurt during and after
4/5/00	20 minutes	Leisurely	More pain, some panic
4/7/00	20 minutes	Leisurely	Hurt during and after, less fear
4/9/00	20 minutes	Leisurely	Hurt during and after
4/10/00	20 minutes	Leisurely	Losing hope, want to quit
4/12/00	20 minutes	Leisurely	A lot of pain, discouraged
4/14/00	20 minutes	Leisurely	Felt better after, some hope

After several more weeks, Tom saw that leisurely walking really didn't make his back any worse. He decided at that point to increase the duration and intensity of his walking:

5/15/00	30 minutes	Fast	Tired, sore, not too worried
5/17/00	30 minutes	Fast	Tired, sore, but okay
5/19/00	30 minutes	Fast	Less tired, more pain, calm

PAIN VERSUS SUFFERING

Distinguishing between pain and suffering to alleviate distress

Many patients tell us, "Your program may work for others, but I've pushed myself before, and it made *me* worse." Having experienced this, they are naturally reluctant to continue doing things they associate with pain. It is important to take a look at what science has learned about pain to help you to continue activities.

The prevailing view in medicine until relatively recently was that pain is a simple physical process—an injury to the body stimulates nerves that transmit a signal to the brain, causing us to feel pain. It was thought to be very straightforward, like pulling on a rope to ring a bell. In the last few decades, however, scientists have found that pain is actually quite complex—it turns out that the degree of pain we feel is only loosely tied to how badly we are injured. All sorts of other factors dramatically influence how much pain we feel. (Recall how powerfully placebos can relieve pain.) Of all these factors, research shows that fear is the most crucial. It seems to open a sort of "gate," which causes pain sensations to be felt more intensely in awareness.

In dealing with chronic back pain, fear plays an even more important role than it does with other types of pain. We've told you how anxiety produces pain, but it also opens the gate, which causes pain signals from the muscles to be amplified once they arrive at the brain. This makes us experience the pain more strongly.

More support for the idea that "simple" pain is a complex phenomenon can be found in the recent work of researchers at Oxford University. They reported that brain scans of individuals who had volunteered to be subjected to (harmless) pain (as research subjects) showed that anticipating physical pain and actually experiencing it activated differing areas of the brain. The study was motivated by a desire to assist in treatment of people experiencing chronic pain, since other research had indicated that the anticipation of pain was often worse than the pain itself for these individuals.

Our interpretation of pain sensations has a big impact on how disturbing they are to us. When we experience a pain in our body that we believe to be harmless, we find it much easier to tolerate than pain that we view as dangerous. As we mentioned, gas pains or cramps can be agonizing, but we tolerate them readily because we think of them as harmless. Likewise, if we trust that the pain will be short-lived, our tolerance increases markedly. If we go out in cold weather without adequate clothing, we can tolerate the discomfort remarkably well, as long as we know that we will be inside again in a few minutes. Pain can be very disturbing, however, if we fear that it means our condition is worsening and it will disable us.

Most people with chronic back pain eventually come to interpret pain sensations in just this sort of negative way. Because the pain has been so burdensome, we do not expect it to be short-lived and harmless. Then even moderate discomfort can make us jump to dire conclusions.

One very important distinction is the difference between the sensation of pain itself and *suffering*. This is not something we are typically aware of. Take a moment now to attend to sensations in your body. Do you feel any discomfort? If so, how would you describe it? Are the sensations aching? dull? sharp? Are they solid or do they throb? tingle? vibrate? Do they stay exactly the same from moment to moment or do they vary a bit? These ever-changing sensations make up "pain."

Suffering includes all of the so-called aversion reactions we have *in response* to pain. These may involve negative thoughts, such as *I hate this, here it is again, this will never get better,* and many of the other emotional reactions that we discussed. It also involves the physical cringing we go through when pain sensations are annoying—bracing the body, tensing our muscles, wincing, and grimacing. It is easy to see these aversion reactions on our faces—it is the very look that we recognize in pictures as a person in pain. Typically, when people "push" themselves "through" pain, their bodies react this way. As you practice paying attention to pain, you may notice that your aversion reactions are much stronger when you worry that the pain is dangerous or will continue. By focusing your attention on the present, you can learn to relax these responses and make the pain much easier to bear.

Many formally established pain management techniques concentrate on learning to relax aversion responses. It is fascinating to note also that, under hypnosis, people can tolerate intense pain—sometimes even that of major surgery. Patients are not unconscious during these experiences—they are deeply relaxed and not resisting the pain.

FOCUSING ON THE PRESENT

Using the attitude of mindfulness to work with pain

Maria, a woman in her mid-fifties, had been suffering with back pain for most of her adult life. At times she had been completely disabled. She lived near the beach and used to love taking long walks. She felt depressed about the loss of this pleasure, but when she tried to resume the walks, her muscles tightened up after only a few minutes and she'd be in serious pain for the next day or two. She felt completely discouraged and wanted to give up.

We decided that the best way to tackle the fear of walking was to walk with Maria and talk her through the pain by cultivating a mindful attitude. As the walks began, she was asked merely to describe the sensations in her body. She started by noticing the feeling of the ground underfoot, the air on her face, the clouds, the trees, and the buildings. As the pain came on, she began paying attention to the sensations of the muscles tightening. Instead of trying to make these sensations go away, she simply noticed the burning, aching, and tingling. When thoughts of damaging herself or becoming trapped in worse pain arose, Maria continued taking note of those thoughts and returning her attention to the sensations of the moment.

She initially feared and fought against the pain, but as she practiced, the sensations changed. By continuing to observe them, she found that her fear decreased and she was able to walk farther. Up until now she had panicked whenever the pain reached a certain intensity.

One of the best antidotes to anxiety about pain is to shift our attention toward the present moment. This is much easier said than done, because we all have a powerful tendency to think about the future. When we experience pain, we start thinking about how long it will last. With chronic back pain, these thoughts can be hair-raising.

It can be enormously reassuring to discover that in fact *all* fear and anxiety involves thinking about the future. This may sound odd at first, but we do not actually fear what is occurring at this moment—we fear what will come next. This is true even when current circumstances are terrible. People who have been in serious accidents report that upon becoming conscious, even if they were in great pain, they became preoccupied with what was *going* to happen to them. Will I die from my injuries? Will I be crippled? No matter what our situation, the mind tends to move toward the future.

Watch your thoughts about your back pain. Notice how many of them are future oriented. Most people find that they are always thinking about the future, often with a good deal of worry.

Because of this powerful inclination, bringing our attention back to the present takes patient practice. A variety of methods can support us in this effort. Most of them involve repeatedly returning our attention to a single focus, such as a repeated word or phrase or a sensation in the body.

The kind of present-centered attention that these techniques develop is often called *mindfulness.* It can assist you in reclaiming the things that you gave up because of pain. Like Maria, you can practice mindfulness by trying to bring your attention to the present when you engage in your chosen activity. If you are walking every day, try to notice the feelings of the ground under your feet, the look of your surroundings, and the feel of the air. You will probably find that your mind wanders pretty quickly. As this happens, just bring your attention back to the here and now. Pain may arise. Try again to notice your future-oriented anxious thoughts: Am I pushing myself too hard? Is this a bad idea? Again, simply take note of these thoughts and bring your attention back to the present.

As you learn to accept the spectrum of present sensations, your fear and aversion to the pain will diminish, and you will be able to widen your range of activity.

In chapter 12 you will find detailed instructions for facilitating mindfulness. If you find that pain and/or anxious thoughts make it difficult for you to resume activity, or find yourself distracted, try these elaborated directions.

TRYING TOO HARD

How overexertion in self-treatment can become a problem

When you use mindfulness in this way to work with pain, you are actually applying two opposite strategies at the same time. On the one hand, you are being quite active—taking control of your life and facing fears by tackling activities that you have avoided. On the other hand, you are being uncommonly passive—simply observing pain in the moment without trying to make it go away. For those recuperating from chronic back pain, figuring out when to be actively striving and when to be receptively accepting is a constant challenge.

Most of us learn early in life that it is necessary to work hard to accomplish our goals. We live in a time when control is prized above all else—our heroes achieve success and power by pursuing them single-mindedly. Even *alternative* medicine touts gaining control over your body. This sort of goal-oriented attitude often works very well, and most successful people rely on it.

Nonetheless, many tasks are actually best accomplished by not trying too hard to achieve a particular outcome. When we try too hard to make our body or mind do our bidding, the tension we generate can get in the way of optimal functioning.

For example, trying to force yourself to fall asleep is usually a losing proposition. Most of us have had anxious nights when we face important responsibilities the next day. We really want to have a good night's sleep. Unfortunately, the harder we try to fall asleep, the more agitated and wakeful we become. This makes us more concerned about being tired, and the night becomes miserable. It is only by giving up on the goal of sleeping that we can relax and fall asleep naturally.

The same thing can be observed in sports. When we try too hard to perform well, our fearfulness creates tension, which, paradoxically, interferes with performance. Successful athletes talk about being in the "zone," during which they are alert and attentive but not self-conscious about their performance. At these times they find that their body moves with effortless grace, and performs well.

Figuring out when to use our will, versus when to let go, is central to breaking the back pain syndrome. A goal-oriented attitude is very handy for constructing a schedule for resuming activities and for sticking to it. It is not useful, however, for dealing with the pain itself. Most chronic back pain sufferers become counterproductively goal oriented in trying to reduce their pain.

It is far better to view the pain itself as uncontrollable—like the weather. This means letting go of the whole gigantic, and ultimately fruitless, project of trying to figure out which actions, chairs, mattresses, and physical treatments seem to make it better or worse. Most of us with chronic back pain become a bit like people who are certain that sacrifices to the gods and avoiding taboos have produced rain for their crops. In effect, we only imagine that we are controlling the pain by our custom-designed rituals of rest and avoidance. The pain may be temporarily diminished, but this relief is largely the result of our belief in these interventions.

Trying too hard can also make our attempts at mindfulness difficult. As you begin to bring your attention to the here and now, you may find that overexertion causes it to wander more. You may think, *My mind is wandering too much*, or, *I'm just no good at being mindful.* We become caught in the preposterous dilemma of being ordered to relax.

The solution involves being open-minded and kind to ourselves. If we take our walk and our mind goes to future-oriented anxiety, we allow this to happen but come back to the present. If our back starts to hurt more, we simply return to the present. If we think that we are no good at this, we do the same. The goal is to try to accept all of these occurrences and continue with our efforts. This is very different from our usual tendency to drive ourselves.

EXPANDING AND REWARDING ACTIVITY

Moving toward the full resumption of life

After several weeks of regularly pursuing a single pleasurable activity, most people will have noticed that their pain varies. Many reach a point where they feel they can continue the first activity without much concern because they have really come to know that it won't make things worse. The next step is to increase the intensity and duration of the activity to the level you would choose if you had no concerns about back pain whatsoever. This should be done at a pace that allows both your body to get into shape and your fears to remain at a tolerable level.

Once you reach your optimum level with an activity, it is time to work with the next one you circled on your "Lost Activities" chart. This might be something a bit more intimidating, but it should still be inherently pleasurable and possible to repeat three or more times per week. If you have grown to fear sitting or standing, pursue these for longer periods. The rest of the assignment is the same as with the first activity: Repeat it at a fixed intensity and duration on a regular, frequent schedule; try to maintain an open attitude toward the pain as it arises; watch the coming and going of anxious thoughts; and take note of moments in which the pain does not seem to get worse.

The program continues along these lines, adding pleasurable pastimes that were previously abandoned one by one. Some people like to get into a cold swimming pool gradually, starting at the shallow end. Others prefer to dive into the deep end right away. As long as you don't overtax your heart and lungs, suddenly overexert neglected muscles, or frighten yourself unnecessarily, you should feel free to move at your own pace. Most people find that their pain is not made substantially worse as they progress. We begin to appreciate the fact that our lack of control over the comings and goings of the pain does not preclude living our lives the way we wish to.

When you have regained most of the pleasurable pursuits you once abandoned, it is time to take on less pleasant but desirable activities. This can be more difficult, since our inner motivation to pursue them is often weaker and our fears can be greater.

HOW FAR TO GO?

Finding the right balance of activity

At some point in working your way through the chart, you may wonder if it is wise to resume each and every one of the activities. After weeks, months, or years of behaving like a person with a "bad back," figuring out how much is enough can be confusing. When is an activity too difficult? We have found that the best general principle is, *Try to act like a normal person.*

If your back pain hasn't lasted too long, you will be able to remember what your life was like before it began. The goal at this point is to return to that level of functioning. If you used to be athletic, try to return to that level of activity. If you were socially active, try to return to that. Remember, the goal is to reclaim your life. The pain will go away on its own.

If your problems have been around for a long time, you may have to turn to others to figure out how to behave. What exactly would normal people of your age, background, athletic conditioning, and life circumstance do? Would they go for a car ride? Would they go for a long walk? Out to dinner? Try to imagine yourself as a person without a bad back and behave accordingly.

FREEDOM FROM MECHANICAL AIDS

Liberating yourself from a counterproductive dependence

Many people suffering from chronic back pain turn to mechanical devices to ease their pain or promote the "healing" of their backs. Often these are originally prescribed by health care professionals. Other times we purchase them in response to advertisements or advice from fellow sufferers. The gadgets include special pillows, back braces and bandages, special chairs and mattresses, "orthotic" shoe inserts, and neck supports. While they may offer some immediate relief, in the long run these devices compound our difficulties by making us think of ourselves as "injured" and interfering with normal movement.

Once you have had success in expanding your range of activities, it is time to begin putting aside mechanical devices. For some people, giving up these aids can be difficult. We may worry that the pain will grow worse if we stop using them or that we will reinjure ourselves.

If you have been using one of these devices, try to let go of it using the same principles that you used to resume activities. Pick the one that you imagine would be easiest to give up. If it is not too frightening to you, try abandoning the device entirely for several weeks. If this feels like too big a step, begin to lay it aside according to a schedule you choose in advance. To make progress, it is important that you put aside the device at least several times each week for a significant period of time.

It is again important to use your schedule rather than your pain level as the basis for using or not using the device. If you put it aside long enough, you will eventually find times in which your pain level rises and falls whether or not you are using the device. This will begin to break your conditioned fear. You may wish to keep a written record of the times you don't use it and your emotional reactions. This will help you to develop certainty that the device is not necessary.

When you notice that a given schedule of use doesn't appreciably worsen your condition, try reducing your use of the aid further. Continue this process until you no longer use it at all. If you have more than one device, try laying aside a second one once you feel secure about having eliminated the first.

The next chapters will examine the obstacles to resuming activity and becoming free of pain that many people encounter.

CHAPTER 9

THE EMOTIONAL TOLL

THIS CHAPTER EXPLAINS:

- How to handle the negative thoughts about your back that occur throughout the day
- How these thoughts lead to upset feelings, tense muscles, and more pain
- How to manage the fear, frustration, anger, and depression caused by your back pain

GETTING BETTER ALL THE TIME

How people recover from chronic back pain

At this point it is likely that you have had some success in resuming your life, and your pain is, at least, not significantly worse. The remaining recuperation period is different for everyone. For most people, taking the steps we have been discussing leads to the recovery cycle illustrated on page 85. This builds confidence, and eventually you start engaging more fully in life. This, in turn, leads to still further feelings of hope, safety, and well-being. You'll notice at first that a few minutes went by without feeling or thinking about pain. Eventually an hour passes without difficulty, and then an afternoon. These periods gradually come more often and last longer, until back pain is no longer at the center of your life. Sometimes this whole process happens very rapidly.

Usually, however, the process is not so seamless. Your confidence grows, is lost, and then develops again. Your pain level may rise and fall many times as you gradually recover. Most people have to experience a number of these episodes to learn that each time the pain eventually lessens and passes.

If you find yourself able to resume living normally, and your pain is gradually going away, you need do no more than keep up the good work. For those of you who find yourselves mired, however, it is important to take a deeper look at the emotional toll of chronic back pain in your life.

EXAMINING YOUR WORRIES

Taking stock of anxiety and fear

As we have indicated, most chronic pain sufferers notice that they think about their backs much of the time. If this is not clear to you, keep a piece of paper with you. Every time that you notice yourself having a negative thought about your back, make a small mark. See how long it takes to fill up the paper.

It can be difficult to concentrate on anything but your sore back. This leads to an interesting problem that doctors often encounter. It goes by the surprisingly untechnical name of the *just not quite right* syndrome. It has to do with the fact that once people become concerned about a part of their body, they tend to become confused about what "normal" feels like.

Bring your attention to the sensations in your right foot. Notice the very faint tingling sensation that's there. Try to concentrate on it for several seconds, to see exactly what it feels like. You may even notice that the sensation feels a little peculiar. It probably feels slightly different from your left foot. Might there be a problem?

In case our point isn't obvious, it is highly unlikely that anything is wrong with your right foot. It's just that every part of our body sends out sensations continuously. Most of the time we don't notice them. Once we start worrying about a body part, it may never again seem to feel "just right." If you have become accustomed to always checking the condition of your back, you may have forgotten, in this sense, what a "normal" back feels like. This can exacerbate your preoccupation with pain.

Very often, people will become more anxious about their backs when facing an important commitment that may aggravate it. This may be an obligation at work, an important social event, or perhaps a trip away from home. Since we are so concerned, the pain often increases just when we least want it to.

After many years of struggling with severe pain, Carrie finally enjoyed several months during which her back was in pretty good shape. She got up the courage to buy airline tickets for a trip to Europe with her boyfriend. She was excited but feared that the trip would be miserable if her back "went out."

As the day of departure approached, Carrie became more and more worried about her back. It had started acting up a little, and she was afraid that it might get worse. Sure enough, a week before she was scheduled to leave, she woke up and could hardly move.

It took a lot of reassurance to convince her that it was safe to travel, but Carrie finally went. After a couple of days of sight-seeing she began to relax.

Simply observing our patterns of worry can be very effective in managing them. By noticing our anxious thoughts, we have the choice to turn our attention back to whatever else we might be doing at the time, rather than getting stuck in a long chain of worries.

A very successful treatment for anxiety called *cognitive-behavioral therapy* teaches people to notice every time they have one of these automatic negative thoughts. When people do this, they find that they no longer *believe* the thoughts in the usual way. Instead of believing in them, they begin to develop a sense of "There goes my mind again, producing those thoughts." This greatly lessens their effect. It becomes a little like watching a suspenseful movie—we are affected by the story but realize at the same time that it's a film, and thus we have a quite different reaction from what we would experience if we actually thought someone was being pursued by a shadowy figure with a knife.

In order to disrupt the cycle, notice the negative thoughts and feelings that *your* pain and mind produce. Depending upon your circumstances, these may include concerns about carrying out specific activities, as well as larger fears involving work, relationships, your ability to take care of yourself and others, and your ability to enjoy life.

Please take a few minutes to complete the "Concerns About Back Pain" form. Take your time, and try to be honest with yourself.

All of the concerns listed in this exercise can be a source of distress. Merely noticing the pervasiveness of these thoughts can help you understand how they affect your pain.

It may seem silly at first, but if your worries about the pain are holding you back, *talk to yourself.* Research has shown that just silently repeating to ourselves the reassuring truth about our concerns reduces stress and helps us to face fear. Rereading earlier chapters of this book, and reminding yourself that you are not damaged and it is safe to exercise, can provide ideas to help. For example, you can repeat to yourself, *It's harmless tension, I can keep going*, or, *I'm just getting scared again, my back is okay.*

Surprisingly, when people begin to resume normal life and pay less attention to their pain, they sometimes feel *more* anxious instead of less. Rather than concentrating our attention on managing pain, we may well encounter more directly the fears that helped to produce it.

Anxiety symptoms can come in many forms. In addition to the worries we've been discussing, some people feel "free-floating" generalized anxiety—restlessness, difficulty concentrating, and feelings of tension.

CONCERNS ABOUT BACK PAIN

The following concerns are often voiced by people struggling with chronic back pain. Read each one and rate how true it is for you. Circle the number at the right that matches your feeling. Skip any items that don't apply to your situation.

0 *Not at all* / 1 *A little bit* / 2 *Moderately* / 3 *A great deal*

The Pain Itself	
My back pain will never get better.	0 1 2 3
I'll never really be happy because of my pain.	0 1 2 3
I'll never feel whole again because of my pain.	0 1 2 3
I won't be able to bear the pain.	0 1 2 3
Work or School	
My pain will interfere with my ability to study, earn a living, or advance in my career in the future.	0 1 2 3
Social Relationships	
I worry about keeping up friendships because of the pain.	0 1 2 3
My pain cuts me off from social activities.	0 1 2 3
I can't have regular sex because of my back pain.	0 1 2 3
My partner will tire of me because of my pain.	0 1 2 3
People won't like me because my back pain makes me irritable and unpleasant.	0 1 2 3
I won't find a romantic partner because of my pain.	0 1 2 3
Family Life and Plans	
I am not being a good parent because of my pain.	0 1 2 3
It is difficult for me to play with my children because of my pain.	0 1 2 3
I am less tolerant at home because of my pain.	0 1 2 3
I don't have children, but I worry that I won't be able to be a good mother or father someday because of my pain.	0 1 2 3
Interests and Activities	
I miss the activities I've given up.	0 1 2 3
I worry that I'll never again be able to enjoy these.	0 1 2 3
Life has lost some of its meaning because of my back pain.	0 1 2 3

The highly intense anxiety episodes that we discussed earlier—panic attacks—are quite common in people who have struggled with back pain. You may recall that they involve a cycle of intensifying anxiety, in which the fear of our own fight-or-flight reaction can rapidly become completely overwhelming. People sometimes feel they would prefer back pain to panic attacks, but panic attacks can be managed.

You may well be able to work with them the same way that you work with your back pain. Recognize and remind yourself that the sensations are harmless. If you can manage to not fight them, they will eventually pass. Many people find that the mindfulness exercises that we detail later can help them to tolerate the bodily distress of panic attacks and other anxiety states.

Should you find that your anxiety is debilitating, it is a good idea to seek professional assistance. Psychotherapy, as described in the next chapter, can be very effective in resolving anxiety problems. In conjunction with psychotherapy, medications may be appropriate for some people (see appendix 2 for more information).

AGGRAVATION

Frustration and anger in the struggle with back pain

Continually grappling with the issues that we have been discussing can lead to the frustration, anger, depression, and exhaustion outlined in chapter 6. Everyone's emotional responses are a bit different, depending on the nature of the pain and how exactly it affects us. Again, looking at your own reactions is essential to breaking the pain cycle.

Has your struggle with chronic back pain been frustrating? Do you feel that no matter what you do, your back keeps hurting? Has this been a harder problem to cope with than others? If you are reading this book, the answer to these questions is probably "Yes."

Even short bouts of back pain make people feel frustrated. We have found that for many people, chronic back pain is the first serious life problem they can't solve. For reasons that we will outline later, many people who develop chronic back pain are competent, "can do" types who are generally quite good at tackling problems. They don't give up easily. If you are such a person, the unsuccessful search for a solution to your pain has probably been extremely frustrating.

Stacey had overcome many obstacles in her life. She grew up poor, with a tough, demanding mother. She had learned early in life to fight for what she wanted and worked her way up to being vice president of a large company. She was good at taking charge and very hard-working.

When the local doctors weren't able to help with her back pain, she pursued well-known experts. She sometimes flew halfway across the country to see them. With each attempt her hopes would rise, only to be dashed again when the pain returned. By the time she came to see us, she had spent over $50,000 of her own money on a fruitless search for relief. Nothing had worked, and she was frustrated beyond measure.

Many years ago, scientists studying emotions asked the question "What causes anger?" While there are several answers to this, one clear cause of anger is frustration. There have been many studies in which people are put in intentionally frustrating situations—sooner or later they start to lose their cool.

Ask yourself how you have dealt with your frustration. Have you noticed yourself becoming angry? Have you felt annoyed at the health care professionals who haven't helped? Are you angry with yourself for "injuring" yourself in the first place or not "taking care" of your back properly? Do you become annoyed at your children or spouse for wanting you to do things while you hurt? Do you get irritable at work when additional demands are placed on you? Are you ever angry at nature, fate, or God for putting you through this? Do you become jealous of others without back pain? Are you angry about all the time you've lost? Are you irritated by suggestions (such as those in this book) that you can do something yourself to end the pain? These sorts of feelings are very common and very understandable.

When you feel irritated or angry, do you take it out on others or hold it in? If you take it out on others, do they become hurt or angry in response? Does this make things worse? If you contain it, does this leave you feeling continually annoyed and tense?

Research shows that significant costs are incurred in trying to control our anger by pushing it out of our mind or denying it. It tends to turn into depression or free-floating anxiety and contributes to various health problems. It is therefore important to examine how you handle angry feelings about your back and whether they might be making an appearance in disguised ways. Do you ever find yourself apprehensive for no apparent reason? Do angry thoughts ever come into your mind when you least expect them? Are you sometimes surprised by angry or violent dreams?

Most of us have difficulty managing our angry feelings, especially when we don't feel they're justified. Very often the anger we feel when suffering through chronic back pain comes from our frustration, and we don't feel right about blaming others for it. This can make the feelings especially tough to deal with.

We will return to the topic of working with anger later and give you a number of tools for managing it.

DEPRESSION

Further long-term consequences of the struggle

We saw in chapter 6 that depression may result from suppressing anger. Depression also comes from learned helplessness—being trapped in pain. Chronic back pain thus often leads to depression. Its symptoms are both mental and physical.

Does your back pain make you feel sad, empty, or tearful? Do you ever feel hopeless or in despair about your back? Do you feel inadequate as an employee, friend, parent, or romantic partner since developing chronic back pain? Do you blame yourself for your back pain problem? Have you lost interest in life's pleasures? Do you ever feel that life is not worth living because of your pain?

Do you easily lose your appetite or eat to excess? Do you find it difficult to sleep or find that you sleep too much? Do you often feel fatigue or experience a lack of energy? Do you have difficulty concentrating or making decisions? Have your lost your usual sexual responsiveness? There can be many causes for any of these symptoms, but when several of them occur together, they usually mean that you are depressed.

Depression takes different forms in different people. You may be sad, or agitated and irritable. One of the worst things about depression is that it can undermine our sense of deserving help with our problems. This is further reinforced by our culture, which tends to see depression as a moral failure rather than a perfectly understandable problem.

When we are depressed, it can be hard to think clearly. Many scientific studies have shown that when suffering from chronic back pain, people think very negatively. We *catastrophize,* imagining the worst-possible scenario and believing that it will really happen. We remember discouraging moments much more vividly than positive ones. We expect failure. Often we have unrealistically self-critical thoughts, such as *I'm worthless if I can't work.* We may even begin to think that we are being punished by God.

Ironically, learning about the true causes of the pain can add to our self-criticism. Many people, understanding that chronic back pain is related to stress, get down on themselves in a whole new way. They blame themselves for being too stressed in the first place or for not handling their emotions better.

For many people, depression begins to lift as soon as they resume activity and find, to their surprise, that they are not crippled. For others, it is necessary to examine the depressive thoughts directly. In the same way that noticing worries helps, noticing depressive thoughts can loosen their grip on us. Take note of how often catastrophic or self-critical thoughts enter your mind. See if you seem to focus on the negative rather than the hopeful. Notice your expectations of failure. You can't force yourself to stop having depressive thoughts, but you will gain perspective and balance by merely observing them.

As you observe your thoughts, be kind to yourself. In the course of getting better, almost everyone feels, *I can't believe I didn't realize this sooner! How could I have gotten myself into such a mess?* We all develop chronic back pain through a chain of completely natural reactions. It is not a sign of mental illness or stupidity.

Sometimes depression becomes so deep that people grow exhausted and don't have the energy to pursue their recuperation. Depression has its own negative cycle in which our life becomes objectively worse because we neglect our relationships and our job. You may feel desperate. If this leads to suicidal thoughts, and especially if you find yourself making suicide plans, please seek help right away from a qualified mental health professional.

As with anxiety problems, psychotherapy can be very effective in resolving depression. Here, too, medications can have their place. The most commonly used medications are the antidepressants discussed in appendix 2.

In the next chapter we'll look at stressors other than back pain itself, and the long-established ways of handling difficult feelings that can promote back pain.

CHAPTER 10

THINK PSYCHOLOGICALLY

THIS CHAPTER EXPLAINS:

- **How excessive emotional control generates stress**
- **The stressful effects of changes in your life**
- **How these stressors can make your pain even worse**
- **How to work with them**
- **Ways that friends and family can support your recuperation**

Concerns about back pain and its effect on our life are an important source of stress for almost everyone suffering from chronic back pain. For some people, however, other concerns also feed the syndrome in a big way.

It may be difficult to know at first if these other issues

are part of your pain problem. If your pain resolves quickly after you resume normal activity, you may not need to explore this. On the other hand, if your pain doesn't seem to be diminishing, or if you suffer at some point from other stress-related maladies, read further. There is then a good chance that your life situation and/or the ways you've learned to handle emotion are contributing to your stress and pain.

Some people expect, when we raise this topic, that we are going to ask them to spend years discussing their childhood, demand that they change their whole personality, or force them to wallow in depressing issues. Actually the process isn't nearly so involved or unpleasant.

KEEPING FEELINGS UNDER CONTROL

The role of inhibited emotion in chronic back pain

While our emotional reactions to back pain play a big part in most chronic back problems, our overall style of managing emotion can be important, too. From early in life we experience a spectrum of feelings, including joy, sadness, anger, fear, longings for closeness, and desires for sensual or sexual pleasure. Every family and culture deals differently with these basic emotions.

If our feelings are met with disapproval when we are young, we learn to suppress them. Sometimes, in order to accomplish this, we try to stop feeling the emotion altogether. For example, if we are told that it is wrong, impolite, or immature to express anger, we may try not to feel angry toward others. If we are taught that it is wrong to cry or appear weak, we may try not to feel sad. We can become remarkably adept at pushing away unwelcome feelings by the time we reach adulthood. We also develop ways of dealing with emotions by observing and interacting with others. Even if nothing is said to us directly, we usually learn to inhibit our own feelings when we are around others who don't express emotions.

Many people learn to block troublesome feelings out of consciousness entirely. This process, which psychologists call *repression,* happens automatically without our knowing about it. Thus when we ask a person who is repressing anger if he or she feels angry, and they answer "No," the person isn't being dishonest. While we can be very good at doing this, repression is never completely successful. Emotions continue to influence our behavior, and our bodily processes, even if they escape our notice entirely.

At certain times, and in certain situations, repressing unwanted thoughts and feelings is useful or even essential. When we go through very difficult periods, repressing thoughts and feelings, for a time, can allow us to function without becoming overwhelmed. This response is not without its costs, however, if it continues over long periods of time. The tendency to keep emotions out of mind can have all sorts of negative effects on our bodies.

Freud noticed that when we are repressing anger we may notice slips of the tongue in which an angry word or gesture leaks out. Very often we will find ourselves anxious or tense for no apparent reason when we are unconsciously angry. When a feeling we have blocked out gets aroused by an event in our life, it threatens, in a sense, to come into our minds. The fear that the unwanted feeling will cause trouble activates our fight-or-flight response.

As we noted earlier, recent research has shown that suppressing anger contributes to many stress-related problems. Repressing anger can play a particularly important role in chronic back pain. When we repress an unwanted feeling, we unconsciously fear that the emotion may pop into our heads or we may find ourselves becoming agitated about many little things. Scientists have discovered that anxiety problems occur most often in people who don't express negative emotions and who like to control their emotions in general. One highly relevant study shows that people with chronic back pain who usually suppress anger have significant increases in back muscle tension when provoked. In this way, the anxiety caused by repressed feelings can feed into the chronic back pain syndrome.

This explains something that often confuses people with back pain: "Why is it sometimes worse in the middle of the night or first thing in the morning, when I'm not using my back muscles and I should be relaxed?" Often the answer is that feelings we push aside during the day come out at night when our guard is down and cause tension. It's the same reason that we may go to bed calm but awaken with a violent nightmare; or learn from our dentist that we are grinding our teeth at night.

Our clinical experience suggests that back pain often comes on, or worsens, when our anger is provoked.

Mark was a very hardworking, likable lawyer. He had grown up in a religious family that emphasized the importance of serving others and turning the other cheek in the face of aggression.

He had been disabled by chronic back pain for several years. He went through many tests and treatments, but nothing helped. Finally, after realizing the true nature of his problem, he was gradually able to return to work. Once back at the office, he began to observe that his pain varied a great deal over the course of a single day. For reasons he couldn't understand, he noticed that his pain increased on several occasions after meeting with his law partners.

Mark didn't like to think of himself as an angry person. When asked to think about it, though, he began to realize that he was annoyed *at the managing partner in his firm. He usually ignored Mark's opinions and had given him an unfair deal when he first joined the practice.*

While it took several weeks, Mark eventually realized that he hated the guy. He'd never admitted it to himself or anyone else. It suddenly dawned on him that his disabling back pain actually began shortly after beginning to work with him.

We can allow ourselves to *feel* difficult emotions without expressing them. It is not necessary to scream at the policeman giving us a traffic ticket or break down crying in the boss's office. Discretion does not actually require repression of feelings. It merely calls for making informed judgments about when to convey them to others.

Psychologists and others have long observed that particular ways of dealing with feelings tend to produce predictable body postures. Some researchers who studied these patterns have concluded that we actually tense certain muscles *as a means of* repressing feelings.

Imagine that you are very sad but trying not to show it. Do you notice how you tighten certain muscles of the face, chest, and belly to hold back the tears?

Each emotion is held back by its own muscle groups. Most of us know this intuitively. When people speak of "steeling" themselves against a feeling, they are describing the way we tense muscles to fight off emotions. If we continually try to block certain feelings, these muscles remain continually tense. The process can also occur in reverse. If we stretch or deeply massage these muscles, sometimes held-back feelings will come out.

This tensing of muscles to hold back emotions is another factor advancing chronic back pain. The repression of unwanted feelings augments chronic back pain both by the generating of overt anxiety and tension when the feelings threaten to surface and by the chronic tightening of muscles that is required to avoid these feelings.

EXAMINING OTHER SOURCES OF STRESS

Understanding the role of life events in your pain

Many things can arouse the negative emotions we have been discussing. In general, all life events and situations that involve *change* create emotional stress. It is important to identify those that may be affecting you. Here are some of the events that scientists have found to be the most stressful. Notice that the list includes both positive and negative situations:

Death of a friend or loved one
Marital separation or divorce
Personal injury or illness
Getting married
Being fired at work
Marital reconciliation
Retirement
Pregnancy
Sex difficulties
Changing jobs
Getting a mortgage
Child leaving home
Trouble with relatives
Beginning or ending school
Moving
Other changes in daily routines
Taking a vacation
Christmas

Looking at this list may give you some ideas. If you have experienced some of these events, think back to how you felt. How did you handle the feelings? Did you keep them to yourself? Did you talk to others?

It is useful to realize that it is not only events themselves but how we experience them that determines how difficult they will be for us. Thus for one person changing jobs or getting married may be relatively easy, while for another it may be pretty traumatic. To recover from chronic back pain, it is important to identify the events that are most intense for you.

Take a moment now to fill out "Coping with Emotions." In the first column, list everything that comes to mind that may have been emotionally stimulating recently. This can include little things, like being overcharged at a restaurant, or larger matters, like a serious argument with your spouse. They may involve ongoing problems, like having too many responsibilities and not enough time. They may be things that make you happy, angry, sad, afraid, lonely—or provoke any other feeling. In the second column, fill in the emotion that you felt in response. In the third column, circle how strong the feelings were. Leave the fourth column, "How I Dealt with the Emotion," blank for now.

It is important to try to include a full range of your emotions. We don't like some of our emotional responses, either because they are too painful or because we are ashamed of them. Most of us, at some point in our lives, struggle with embarrassing feelings of inadequancy, dependency, helplessness, conflict about sexuality, fears about aging, guilt, shame, or humiliation in addition to simpler feelings of joy, anger, sadness, and fear. As we will see shortly, our unwanted emotions are the most important ones to address in order to recover from chronic back pain.

Now look at the list. Which areas of your life seem to have the most difficult emotions associated with them? Which are the strongest emotions? We will discuss how to work with these shortly.

GETTING TO KNOW YOU

Exploring our everyday style of dealing with emotions

Now go to the fourth column of the "Coping with Emotions" exercise. Make a note of how you managed each feeling that you wrote down. Did you express it? Did you keep it to yourself? Did you try to hold on to it so it wouldn't fade? Did you try to make it go away?

COPING WITH EMOTIONS

EVENT:	EMOTIONS IT BRINGS UP (HAPPY, SAD, ANGRY, WORRIED, FRUSTRATED, ETC.):	STRENGTH OF FEELING: 1 = MILD 2 = MODERATE 3 = STRONG	HOW I DEALT WITH THE EMOTION:
FAMILY:		1 2 3	
		1 2 3	
		1 2 3	
		1 2 3	
		1 2 3	
		1 2 3	
SOCIAL/ FRIENDS:		1 2 3	
		1 2 3	
		1 2 3	
		1 2 3	
		1 2 3	
		1 2 3	
WORK:		1 2 3	
		1 2 3	
		1 2 3	
		1 2 3	
		1 2 3	

		1 2 3	
HEALTH:		1 2 3	
		1 2 3	
		1 2 3	
		1 2 3	
OTHER:		1 2 3	
		1 2 3	
		1 2 3	

Next look for patterns. Do you find that some feelings appear more often than others? This may mean that you are more comfortable with certain emotions than others. Are there some feelings that you typically push away and others that you are more likely to express? We are all different in how we handle feelings, and recognizing your unique pattern of coping is important.

The feelings we feel readily, and find it easy to accept or express, do not generally add to chronic back pain. These emotions typically arise and pass away easily, leaving little residue of tight muscles. Like a young child, we feel these feelings fully, express them immediately, and let them pass.

The feelings that do increase chronic back pain are the ones that we don't recognize or express readily and those that we try to push away. These often produce anxiety and tension.

In the exercise, which feelings were missing or appeared infrequently? Take a few minutes to reflect on whether these emotions were always difficult for you or whether there was a time in your life when you learned to suppress or repress them.

In our experience, certain patterns emerge most frequently among people with chronic back pain. For example, many of the people we work with are highly conscientious. They go out of their way to be responsible and not offend others. They arrive on time for appointments, follow through on promises, and rarely express anger. They often strive to be rational and reasonable and feel uneasy in the presence of raw emotion. This personality style has worked well for them. They are understandably concerned that if they act more angrily or selfishly, people will no longer like them.

Closely related to these qualities is a tendency toward perfectionism. Many people we treat feel unusually compelled to be very thorough in their work. They are self-critical and feel guilty or inadequate when they make mistakes. They tend to prefer to suffer themselves rather than make problems for others.

Jamie was, by everyone's account, "a nice guy"—consistently pleasant and helpful. He hadn't always been this way. As a boy, he got into frequent trouble for fighting at school and felt like a misfit.

He had a demanding father who insisted on good behavior, though. By the time he was a teenager, he had begun to conduct himself in an exemplary manner. As an adult he made a point of being on time, eating a healthy diet, and keeping his apartment neatly organized. His reports at work were so complete that his boss used them as a model for training others.

Jamie had suffered from back pain for some time. When we began looking at his emotional life, he noticed that it had become seriously restricted. While he felt lonely sometimes, and was often anxious, he never got angry at anyone and hardly ever felt excitement or joy. Jamie was quick to be understanding of others and rarely blamed them.

Jamie realized that he used to get angry a lot but found that it only caused trouble, and he learned to block out the feeling. While it took some time, he eventually rediscovered his emotions. Anger at his father eventually surfaced, along with feelings of jealousy and longings for closeness. No longer so excessively reasonable, he also began to feel much more alive.

Your particular pattern of handling emotions may well be different. What is important is that you both look at how you've been dealing with your feelings up until now and work toward noticing them more clearly.

DEVELOPING A PSYCHOLOGICAL PERSPECTIVE ON PAIN

Putting your attention in the right place

People often use distraction as a means of avoiding difficult emotion. It may involve "burying" ourselves in a book, spending too much time at the mall, or becoming obsessed with minor decisions. Surprisingly, worrying about our back pain can also serve to distract us. This is a bit complicated. Not only do our concerns about our back pain cause pain directly, but these same concerns can distract us from noticing important underlying emotions, such as anger or sadness, that generate pain. Sometimes the pain appears to persist, in part, *because* it distracts us from thoughts and feelings that we would rather not face.

> *Tim had friends, and dated, but often felt lonely because he didn't have a girlfriend. He felt very hurt and angry when relationships didn't work out. Because of his upbringing, Tim found it hard to express these feelings and didn't even like admitting them to himself.*
>
> *In the course of trying to understand his back pain, Tim began to observe his emotions for the first time. He also began to notice a pattern—whenever something happened in his life that made him sad or angry, he developed physical pain. Once this pain began, his thoughts went to worrying about it, so that he no longer noticed his other feelings. The pattern was most pronounced when a relationship ended.*
>
> *After a while Tim learned to ask, "What might my pain be distracting me from?" He became quite good at recognizing the underlying feelings, and his pain episodes passed much more quickly.*

We are so used to thinking physically—wondering what activity or treatment has made our pain better or worse—that we often forget to ask ourselves what thoughts or feelings may be fueling the changes. By working toward thinking psychologically, we begin to recognize our underlying feelings and prevent preoccupation with pain from undermining our recovery.

When asked to attend to their feelings in this way, some people worry that it will make them "weak." Many people are taught to think that only ineffective people allow themselves to feel upset, whereas strong people are always in control of their emotions. This is a common misunderstanding. One of the early astronauts was asked how he could be so fearless as to go up into space with untested equipment. He replied, "Fearless? I was terrified! Courage isn't being without fear. It's doing what has to be done despite it."

People often say, "What good does it do to think about aggravating things? It only makes matters worse." While it is true that people can get stuck in a pattern of dwelling on negativity, paying attention to what's bothering us is usually advantageous. Our chances of being relaxed in our bodies, and finding solutions to problems, are actually much better if we let ourselves notice the full range of our emotions.

There is a lot of scientific evidence that attending to our feelings helps with stress-related problems in general. People who suffer from panic attacks or periods of anxiety often feel that they come "from nowhere," much as back pain sometimes seems to. Researchers have discovered that these symptoms are actually preceded by events that cause sadness, anger, or fear. The person with the anxiety problem often doesn't notice these other feelings until asked about them. Once their attention is brought to the emotions, the problem begins to fade.

Thinking in this way is really very straightforward. It means regularly taking time to ask, "Is anything bothering me emotionally?" The question is especially important when you feel an increase in back pain. You then think about recent events in your life and turn your attention toward any emotions that you may be experiencing, rather than worrying about overtaxing your back. If this process does not seem to come naturally to you, the next section provides some tools to help.

Once they begin thinking psychologically, many people find it gradually gets easier and becomes natural. They also identify past stressors in their life that probably caused, or at least contributed to, their back problem in the first place. People often realize, in retrospect, that they were under stress from one or more of the life situations listed earlier or from other important changes in their circumstances.

WORKING WITH ANGER

When should *we express it?*

As we have indicated, suppressing anger is particularly problematic for chronic back pain sufferers.

Of all our emotions, anger can be the trickiest to work with. The newspaper is full of stories of its destructive power. We hear conflicting messages about it: "Turn the other cheek," but "Don't let them walk all over you"; "Forgive and forget," but "Stand up for yourself"; and so on. Many of us automatically push the feelings away as a result.

Letting ourselves *feel* anger, even if we don't express it, is the middle ground. It is a good place to begin. Try filling in the blank with the first word that comes to mind: "I resent______." Repeat "I resent______" five or more times, filling in the blank with whatever annoyances you can think of. It doesn't matter if they are big or small, justifiable or not. Most people find that there are scores of things they feel angry or resentful about.

Once you've thought about this, ask yourself if it might be appropriate to express *any* of these feelings. If someone continues to act badly, just noting the anger does little to correct the situation. We often either characteristically hold back our anger, becoming too *passive* or overdo expressing it, becoming too *aggressive.* What works best is often called being *assertive.*

When we are *passive,* we avoid saying what we want, think, or feel. We tend to put ourselves down or be apologetic about expressing ourselves. We let others make choices for us and try to hide our displeasure.

When we are *aggressive,* we say what we want, think, or feel, but at the expense of others. We don't own feelings as our own, but label, judge, or blame others. We talk about how "you" did something wrong, sometimes using threats or trying to "one-up" the other person. We make choices for others.

Assertiveness involves saying what we want, think, or feel, but in direct and effective ways. We talk clearly about what *we* feel, not demanding that others feel the same way or see things as we do. We express interest in understanding the other person's point of view. Tact and humor are used to communicate. We negotiate choices.

If you find yourself feeling angry and being either passive or aggressive, it will be worth your while to practice assertiveness. Sometimes a few well-chosen words or an open conversation with someone we've been angry at can do a lot to ease stress and tension. The guidelines for improving communication that we include under the "Friends and Family" section of this chapter incorporate principles of assertiveness.

When people who suffer from characteristically bottling up even well-justified anger learn of the problematic aspects of that habit, they sometimes presume that those who generally let it out are far better off in life. After all, pop psychology is full of accounts of therapists inducing their patients to scream their upsets and punch pillows. Research suggests that impulsively venting may be fraught with difficulties, too. It indicates that aggressive "blowing off steam" often appears to increase aggression rather than release it.

Solid scientific research shows that practicing assertiveness can do a lot to improve your relationships, reduce the buildup of unexpressed anger, and lower your overall stress level. Even in situations where it doesn't make sense to confront anyone, we can still pay attention to the feeling and perhaps discuss it with an uninvolved person we trust.

It may be best to let go of resentments, in time, if there is nothing that can be done about them. Finding the right time to do that is an art. If we try to let go of angry feelings before we've felt them, they may produce stress symptoms. On the other hand, if we harbor grudges indefinitely, they can add unhappiness to our lives.

INCREASING AWARENESS OF YOUR EMOTIONS

Tools for uncovering and exploring feelings

There are a variety of structured methods that can help you to recognize and cope with emotion more effectively.

MINDFULNESS

We've discussed how cultivating an attitude of mindfulness can help you to bear back pain. The same approach can be applied to emotions. We usually have a tendency to try to hold on to pleasant emotions and get rid of uncomfortable ones. This natural impulse brings on our fight-or-flight response. When we cling to pleasant emotions, we become anxious that we will lose them. When we are trying to get away from unpleasant feelings, we are often agitated. We complicate painful emotions in our rush to avoid them, becoming upset *about* being upset.

The alternative to this involves learning to accept the coming and going of both positive and negative emotions. This is easier said than done, but by accepting them, we become less distressed about the things that bring them on.

What is important in practicing mindfulness is allowing ourselves to feel emotions fully. We can then use our judgment to decide when, where, and how they should be conveyed.

It is easiest to be mindful when alone. Take a few minutes to observe any feelings you may be experiencing right now. Do you notice any sadness? any anxiety? joy? anger? Notice the sensations these emotions generate in your body. Is there tightness? warmth? Is your heart beating quickly? What is your breathing like? Do you feel the emotion in your chest, throat, or belly? Common expressions speak to these sensations: "a heavy heart," "the weight of the world on his shoulders," and "a lump in the throat" are all examples.

Don't try to change the emotions. Watch them come, observe them, and see how they change by themselves. You may notice all sorts of thoughts surrounding them. Bring your attention back to whatever feelings are present. Techniques that can strengthen your capacity for mindfulness appear in chapter 12.

JOURNAL WRITING

A number of studies have shown that writing about the things that upset us can improve health. In one study, asking college students to keep a journal (for four days) about past emotional difficulties reduced their visits to student health services. The writing also produced a measurable enhancement of their immune system. In another study, journal writing produced lasting improvements in asthma and arthritis symptoms. These benefits result from the stress-reducing effects of acknowledging and experiencing painful emotions.

All that you have to do is to set aside fifteen minutes a day to write in a diary. At first, it is best to write every day, for at least several days in a row. After this, it doesn't have to be done daily—even once a week will help. Establish a regular schedule and add sessions any time that something is bothering you. Write someplace where you won't be interrupted.

You can write about any emotional event, though it is especially important to include negative experiences. Be sure to explore hurt, sadness, anger, fear, guilt, and resentment. Try to include your deepest thoughts and feelings, including those that you might not want to express to others. You can keep your writings private.

Try to write continuously, without worrying about spelling, grammar, or even making sense. If you run out of things to say, you can repeat what you have already written.

Don't be concerned if journal writing makes you *more* unhappy at first. This is perfectly natural when we turn our attention toward painful feelings. Most people find that they feel relief and greater contentment after several writing sessions.

Of course, if you are coping with highly traumatic events such as death, divorce, or violence, you won't feel better immediately. Over time, however, writing can help you to get a better perspective and reduce your stress.

SELF-HELP GROUPS

If you have identified a particular problem as the source of a lot of stress in your life, self-help groups can be beneficial. There are community groups for almost every problem you can think of—substance abuse, serious illnesses, death and aging, sexual or physical abuse, and divorce.

Talking to others with similar experiences helps us feel less ashamed of our reactions, since we usually find that other people share them.

Many times we also find that others have found ways to deal with problems that we haven't thought of, which can aid us in discovering our own solutions. Self-help groups are a proven way to tap into the powerful stress-reducing, health-enhancing benefits of positive relationships.

We do not, however, recommend those self-help groups that focus on chronic pain. Most members of chronic pain support groups and chronic pain-related Internet chat rooms believe that their back pain is due to structural damage or disease. They can problematically reinforce your fears about having an incurable disability.

PSYCHOTHERAPY

Many people are reluctant to consult a mental health professional for help. Our society places a very high value on solving one's own problems. Emotional distress is often seen as a sign of failure, and many people therefore avoid seeking help until they are desperate. In some circles people still think that only crazy people need "shrinks."

This is very unfortunate. So many of us live silently and secretly with emotional pain and suffer needlessly from symptoms related to common difficulties. Stress-related problems are rampant in our society, yet for many people the thought of seeing a psychologist, psychiatrist, or other mental health professional is almost unthinkable.

Seeing a mental health professional does not mean that you are emotionally disturbed in any way. A trained professional can help you to understand what is causing your distress and find ways to work with it in a finite amount of time.

There are a variety of therapeutic methods that have something to offer in treating chronic back pain. Some focus more on repressed or suppressed emotions, while others concentrate on overcoming fears and identifying irrational thought patterns that cause anxiety or depression.

Most important in choosing a psychotherapist is finding one with an understanding of stress-related disorders. Some psychotherapists are stuck in the cycle of chronic back pain themselves. These therapists may transmit their own fears, which obviously won't help. Physiatrists, physical therapists, and other medical professionals who encourage their patients to resume full activity can sometimes refer you to appropriate psychotherapists. Many psychotherapists who specialize in behavioral medicine have experience working with chronic back pain from this perspective.

It is also important that you feel comfortable with any psychotherapist you see. You will need to confide in them, and this requires considerable trust. You should discuss any reservations you have at the outset. No one therapist is right for every person, and it may take a little searching to find someone you can work with to best advantage.

FRIENDS AND FAMILY

Getting help from the people you care about and coping with relationship difficulties

As we begin to make progress, our family and friends usually take notice. Depending upon their own attitude about our back problem, and their own orientation toward emotion, they may or may not be of help.

Usually they have seen us go through plenty of ups and downs with our backs. They may be as fearful as we are that we will get worse or never recover. Our back problem is difficult for people who are close to us, too.

Just like us, our friends and family have probably thought that our back pain is due to some sort of damage to our spine. They may encourage us to be careful and not push ourselves. They may volunteer to lift things for us and may plan limited activities so as not to aggravate our condition. While meaning well, our family and friends usually share the belief that our backs are fragile and become overly protective.

This can be even more true if they have had back troubles themselves or have cared for others in pain. Researchers have found that people who become disabled by chronic back pain tend to have a family history of the same problem. Many people may learn to fear their pain in part because they have seen others become disabled.

Just as we have to gradually change our attitude in order to get better, friends and family can best support us by changing theirs.

While it may have been difficult for you to believe that your pain is caused by stress, it may be even more difficult for you to explain this to others. Most of us worry that others either won't believe us or will conclude that we must be emotionally disturbed to have developed such a problem. On top of this, we may worry that our loved ones will blame us for putting them through hell once they understand that the problem could have been resolved earlier.

Michele felt terrible for causing her husband so much trouble with her pain. While he was very supportive, she believed that he really didn't think it was that bad, was secretly angry at her, and thought she should "get over it." His own approach to problems was to tough it out. At the same time, he had been quick to pick up the slack, doing all of the shopping and cleaning.

When Michele began to realize the real cause of her problem, she was both relieved and horrified. Being self-critical to begin with, she was angry with herself for not realizing what was going on sooner. She was sure that once her husband learned the truth, he'd be furious.

Their first conversations were tough, because he didn't understand what she was trying to tell him. Then it began to make sense to him. He was initially annoyed and took on something of an "I told you so" attitude. It wasn't long, however, before he was grateful to have a functional wife back, and their marriage took a turn for the better.

We have found that it is important to let family and friends know that we are no longer so limited by our back pain and to ask them to begin treating us like normal people. For those who might be less understanding, you may want to simply explain that you have learned that increasing movement is not harmful to your back.

One good strategy for getting support is to announce our plans to try new things. Once we declare our intentions, we may feel more reluctant to put off or avoid the challenges we have planned for ourselves.

You may also want to ask the people you trust to stop unknowingly reinforcing your preoccupation with pain. You can ask them to stop inquiring about how your back is doing. Instead you can ask them to commend you when they see you engaging in activity.

For those with whom you can share feelings openly, discussing the relationship between your back pain and emotions can also help. Most people find that as they pay more attention to their feelings, they're tempted to share them. Expressing emotions to important people in our lives also helps us to experience them more clearly.

Depending on your particular background, this may or may not come easily. Of course, both men and women can grow up in families or cultures that "keep a stiff upper lip" and "don't air dirty laundry." Generally, in our society, women get more practice at expressing feelings, because they are encouraged to do so more than men are. Men are often taught to hide emotion, except for perhaps anger, enthusiasm on the playing field, or sexual interest. This can become a real stumbling block for relationships.

One particular type of friendship deserves mention because it can be tricky to handle—friends who are also back pain sufferers. If they aren't ready to consider your new way to solve the problem, they can undermine your progress by repeating warnings about movement and trying to convince you that your back really is damaged. We often see people struggle to maintain these friendships while recognizing that they are problematic. Usually the best solution is to avoid discussing your back problem with them until you are sufficiently active and pain free that their opinions no longer affect you. They will eventually notice that you have gotten better and may even become interested in how you did it.

ENHANCING COMMUNICATION

It probably won't surprise you to hear that back pain can sometimes take a serious toll on intimate relationships. Researchers have found that the spouses of people with chronic back pain themselves become stressed and often depressed. They may be unhappy about our limitations, resentful about taking care of us, and weary of our moods. They can find it hard to deal with sexual difficulties, increased responsibility, and worries about income. This often leads to marital conflict and dissatisfaction. (The good news is that despite these problems, back pain does not lead to increased divorce.)

It's not hard to see how our partner's exasperation might, in turn, increase our own stress level. There's nothing like an argument to turn on our fight-or-flight response. Scientists have even found that stressful encounters with their spouses will make people with chronic back pain give up on physical activity, while positive interactions make it possible for them to do more.

In general, the best way to develop and maintain good relationships is by improving communication. Often this is difficult, since when we are in pain, we may not feel like talking. We may also feel that we don't want to hear about other people's problems. It is nonetheless worthwhile. Here are some guidelines for opening communication channels if you're feeling cut off from people you care about:

- **Pick a good time.** It is best to find an occasion when both you and the other person are relaxed and therefore have the best chance of being open to each other.

- **Ask others what your ordeal has been like for them.** Invite them to share their own frustrations and fears. While it may be painful at first, this will open up communication.

- **Just listen.** Our usual reaction to hearing others' problems is to offer solutions. "Why don't you just______instead?" or "I'm sorry, from now on I'll______" There will be time to find solutions later. It is most important to hear the other person's feelings.

- **Try on their point of view.** We often have difficulty seeing what things are really like for another person. Take some time to imagine being in their shoes and consider what you might feel.

- **Speak directly.** This usually means making "I" statements, such as "I feel______" or "I want______" rather than "You make me feel______" or "You are a______." Try to speak clearly about your own wishes or needs.

- **Be diplomatic.** It may take the other person time to accept what you are saying. Presenting it diplomatically can help.

- **Don't use "shoulds."** Often we're tempted to tell others that they *should* feel or act a certain way. We may say, "You shouldn't feel upset." This is almost guaranteed to make things worse.

- **Avoid blaming or taking blame.** It is usually necessary not to figure out who is at fault, but to understand how each of your actions makes the other person feel. Most tensions are caused by problematic exchanges—not a "right" or "wrong" individual.

- **Allow others time to respond.** It is important to listen to the other person's response, even if he or she is becoming angry or defensive. Once you've taken in what the other person has to say, you can respond directly with your own feelings.

- **Remember the good times.** Sometimes, when we've been through a lot of pain or strife, we forget about the nice parts of our relationships. When trying to communicate more, remember and acknowledge the positive.

As you move forward with the program, you may run into some unexpected pitfalls. We will try to guide you through these in the next chapter.

CHAPTER

11

COMMON PITFALLS

THIS CHAPTER EXPLAINS:

- How to overcome the special challenges posed by other stress-related disorders and seriously disturbing life occurrences
- Other common obstacles and dilemmas

OTHER STRESS DISORDERS

The astounding spectrum of related maladies

Stress can bring on all sorts of physical symptoms. They may predate our back pain or come on after it. These symptoms are unnerving when they occur along with chronic back pain because we may begin to think that we are falling apart. They tend to follow a pattern that is remarkably similar to that of chronic back pain. They may begin with an infection or injury, or they may begin with stress. Sometimes the stress of dealing with back pain itself brings them on. Once they start, we become concerned about the symptom. This activates our fight-or-flight system, which makes the symptom worse. It then causes the same sort of anxiety, depression, frustration, and exhaustion that are common in the chronic back pain syndrome.

As we've mentioned, the most common ones include digestive difficulties, headaches, skin rashes, dizziness, ringing in the ears (*tinnitus*), grinding teeth, anxiety, sleep disturbances, fatigue, sexual performance problems, bladder discomfort, and pain in other muscles or joints. *All of these problems can have varied causes, and you should seek an evaluation from a physician before assuming that stress is the culprit.* Once other causes are ruled out, however, these difficulties can generally be treated much like your back pain.

For a surprising number of people, one of these symptoms may develop just as their back pain subsides. If this happens to you, it probably means that you are under a good deal of stress and may be having difficulty with some emotional issue.

Just as with back pain, solving these problems involves understanding the cause of the symptom, stopping our fight against it, shifting our focus to living normally, and paying attention to other emotional events in our life. Then they will go away on their own.

PAIN IN OTHER MUSCLES OR JOINTS

One of the most common maladies people develop once their back pain subsides is pain in another muscle or joint. Unfortunately, these too are often mistakenly attributed to a structural defect.

> *Jessica had been devastated by her back problem but was on the mend. She was starting to exercise, and life was getting back to normal.*
>
> *One day, while jogging, her knee started to bother her. This made her nervous. When she ran again the next day, the pain was back and felt worse. She figured that something must be irritated, so she stopped jogging for the rest of the week. It made her feel like an old lady.*

> *The next week, the same thing happened.* I just can't win, *she thought.* Just when I was beginning to get my life back together, *this* had to happen. *Her doctor sent her to an orthopedist, who diagnosed* chondromalacia patella—*worn cartilage under the kneecap. He recommended leg exercises and giving up anything that might further wear out her knee. She felt like giving up on living.*

As we mentioned, lots of body parts can develop stress-related pain. Doctors investigate, often find some abnormality, and frequently recommended restricting activity.

In addition to *chondromalacia,* patients walk away from medical visits with ominous-sounding diagnoses such as *arthritis, tendinitis, bursitis, bone spurs, plantar fasciitis, temporomandibular joint syndrome,* and *repetitive strain injury.* If they have several of these problems at once, they may be told that they're suffering from *fibromyalgia.*

It is beyond the scope of this book to examine each of these conditions in depth. Nonetheless, you should know that while they too may begin as acute injuries, *very often* these problems are perpetuated by muscle tension. They are usually best treated by a return to activity and attention to stress. In deciding on a course of action, you will benefit from finding a doctor who understands this. Again, physiatrists, who deal extensively with muscle problems and rehabilitation, are often your best bet.

We see many people for whom the pain travels from place to place every few days or weeks. Each time, if they worry, it tends to stick around; but if they treat it as stress-related muscle pain, it goes away.

SEXUAL PROBLEMS

Concern over physically harming our back, depression, and distraction from the pain itself can reduce our interest in sex. Many people become alarmed if they find that they cannot perform sexually.

> *Carl was a dedicated worker. His job required long hours and carried a great deal of responsibility. His back pain had become intense and*

unremitting. He was newly married, and pleased with his marriage, but he felt anxious and depressed most of the time.

While he initially feared sex because of his back, he now feared that he wouldn't be able to perform. The harder he tried to perform sexually, the more his body failed to respond. He was once exceptionally self-assured but now felt broken.

While this sort of problem can be caused by medications or purely physical conditions, stress is usually to blame. What makes matters worse is that people often feel singularly ashamed of sexual symptoms and are afraid to tell anyone. If this has happened to you, we want to reassure you that it is a widespread problem. Most successful treatments incorporate principles very similar to those of the Back Sense program, if the problem is not due to medication or a purely physical disorder.

It is important to involve our sexual partners in working this out. Often they are also apprehensive about vigorous movement causing injury. This can cause them to inhibit their own sexual response and make us feel more anxious. They need to be reassured.

It is also a good idea to explain to your partner that you are still attracted to him or her, but the pain-related distress sometimes keeps your body from responding in the usual way. Many couples also find it helps to refrain from intercourse for a while and engage in other forms of mutual stimulation, so as to reduce the pressure to perform. Once the pressure is off, our bodies begin to function again. If the problem is persistent, you can consult your doctor.

SLEEP DISTURBANCES

Of all stress-related problems, insomnia is probably the most common in people with back pain. There are a number of factors that lead to this: lack of physical activity during the day, use of medications, anxiety, depression, and the pain itself.

It is not surprising that the body's fight-or-flight system interferes with sleep—if we are in danger, it's a good idea to stay awake. This can result in what researchers call *nonrestorative sleep.* Even if we've managed to fall asleep, we wake up unrefreshed. Though sleep problems typically get better as back pain lessens and activity increases, there are steps you can take to help.

Trying too hard to get to sleep is guaranteed to keep you awake and set up a pattern of bedtime distress. It is therefore *most* important to adopt an accepting attitude toward insomnia, realizing that it is unpleasant but usually not dangerous. With this in mind, the following suggestions can often help:

- **Don't spend a lot of time in bed when you aren't sleeping—don't read in bed, watch television, or lie there worrying about falling asleep.**

- **If you do not fall asleep within fifteen to twenty minutes of going to bed, either**

    1. get out of bed and do something quiet, such as reading in fairly dim light (television is usually a bad idea, as the bright light fools the brain into staying awake); then return to bed when you get sleepy; or

    2. do some meditation or relaxation exercises, described in the next chapter. Meditation can provide some of the same restorative benefits while you are awake.

- **Avoid caffeine, alcohol, and cigarettes late in the day.**

- **Avoid late night exercise, but make sure you are exercising.**

- **Avoid napping for more than thirty minutes during the day.**

- **Try to keep regular times for going to bed and waking up, even on the weekends.**

- **Estimate how many hours you are currently sleeping each night, and spend only that amount of time in bed. This will**

gradually cause a slight sleep deficit, which will make it easier to quickly fall asleep.

If these steps don't help enough, professional guidance and medication can be of assistance.

SPECIAL COMPLICATIONS

Potential traps

In the course of struggling with chronic back pain, special issues sometimes crop up that can make it difficult to pursue recovery. It is rare for any one person to experience all of these, but it is common to find oneself coping with at least one of them. While there are many books completely devoted to each of these problems, we want to offer some brief guidelines here to point you in the right direction.

IDENTITY CRISES: WHO AM I NOW?

Sometimes our sense of self is deeply connected to being physically strong or successful at work. Fearing that we have lost this can make us feel undone, as though our whole identity has been compromised.

Jason had spent his entire adult life working in the shipping industry. He was proud of his work as a pipe fitter and proud to be a father supporting his family. When he was younger, he was the star of his amateur baseball team. He felt popular and well respected, largely because he was a talented athlete.

After his accident, everything changed. He thought that he could no longer bend or lift anything heavy. Because of this he was unable to continue working at the shipyard and began collecting disability payments.

Jason became very depressed. If he couldn't be the kind of worker and breadwinner that he once was, he felt that life wasn't worth living. He couldn't imagine doing any other kind of work. When a counselor suggested that he look into computers, he couldn't stand the idea. It just wasn't him.

As the weeks dragged on, he felt that he didn't know who he was anymore. He started drinking heavily and was irritable with his family. This only made him feel worse about himself.

A remarkable number of people with chronic back pain go through crises like Jason's. Some earn their living using physical strength. Others have relied on physical abilities for their sense of themselves. For some people, being attractive and in shape has always been rewarding. When these things are taken away, we can feel an emptiness and confusion that we may have never faced before. Our self-esteem can plummet. These feelings can become especially overwhelming if you stop working and think of yourself as disabled.

If this happens to you, it may be beneficial to get counseling. These sorts of problems are surprisingly common, and a trained professional can help.

FACING MORTALITY

In a related problem, struggling with chronic back pain often forces people to face their own eventual death. Most of us don't like to think or talk about this. A therapist who conducts workshops on the topic tells a story in which he asks a large audience, "Who here is going to die?" Usually only about a third of the hands go up! Many of us don't actually *see* people die very often. Very old, infirm, or seriously ill people often live away from our communities in special facilities. Television, movies, and advertisements are overflowing with images of youthful vitality. Much of the time our minds are full of plans for a long future.

Chronic back pain can bring about a rude awakening in this regard. After struggling with pain at length, many people begin to notice the fragility of life. Sooner or later bodies give out. Feeling this directly can be shocking and even depressing. Our culture tells us it is "morbid" and "unnatural" to dwell on these matters, and people often feel embarrassed to tell others they are thinking about it.

If you've been troubled by such thoughts, it is best to acknowledge them directly. It can be good to talk with friends or family whom you trust. If you are religious, you may want to speak with your priest, minister, or rabbi.

RELIVING PAST TRAUMA

While not everyone who suffers from chronic back pain has experienced past trauma, a number of studies show that it is remarkably common. A study at a large university's health service showed that 60 percent of women with chronic back pain reported having been sexually abused as children. Far fewer women without back pain had suffered such abuse. Similar statistics can be found for childhood physical abuse and other traumas. People with a number of different stress-related problems are more likely than other people to have suffered through difficult times as a child.

In our work, we often find that this affects how people react to their pain in the present. Sometimes the pain and inability to get help remind us of inescapable pain we once felt. We may try to cope with current pain the way we tried to cope with trauma in the past.

Meg's mother used to scream and beat her. The outbursts were unpredictable, and Meg struggled to find a place to hide in their tiny house. As she got older, she learned to fight back, and this helped her to become resourceful and competent in life.

When Meg's back pain got bad, she became very angry. The pain reminded her of her mother's relentless tirades. She felt as though the pain were "beating on" her, and she couldn't find a way to fight back. She found herself in a state of lonely insecurity that she thought she had left behind with her agonizing childhood.

We often encounter histories of child abuse, early death, hostile divorce, serious illness, war trauma, serious accidents, and rape or other violent crimes.

If you have suffered serious trauma in the past, there is a good chance that it colors your reaction to your back pain. It all depends on the nature of the trauma, your temperament, and your coping strategies.

In general, we counsel becoming more aware of emotion. However, because the intensity of feelings and memories connected to trauma can be so overwhelming, it can be hazardous to try to recover them suddenly. It is important to feel a sense of safety and stability in our life before bringing these things back into awareness.

If you are having difficulty with the effects of past trauma, or suspect that blocked feelings from a trauma are contributing to your stress, it is usually wise to consult with a qualified mental health professional. He or she can help you to evaluate the best way to work with these.

DRUGS AND ALCOHOL

It is not unusual for chronic back pain sufferers to get themselves into trouble by using drugs or alcohol excessively to relieve anxiety, depression, and physical pain.

While medications can have a place in relieving chronic back pain, it is important to evaluate whether they are interfering with your life. This disruption can occur in several ways:

- **Medications themselves can "reward" us for being in pain. This is even more true if we take them "as needed" rather than on a regular schedule. They may feel good or temporarily relieve emotional distress.**

- **It is crucial to remain clearheaded when we tackle the challenge of returning to activity. When our thought processes are clouded by drugs or alcohol, we have difficulty following the program.**

- **Many medicines dampen the intensity of emotions, interfering with our ability to deal effectively with them. In the long run, this increases tension.**

- **Drugs tend to interfere with sleep. While they may help us to fall asleep initially, they can keep us from dreaming normally, which leaves us less well rested.**

- **Alcohol, narcotics, tranquilizers, and sleeping medications can all contribute to depression. They can make you moody or irritable and rob you of the energy necessary to recuperate.**

People generally do better as they come off pain medications. While these medicines may occasionally have a useful role in helping a person function through a *brief* period of acute pain caused by an injury, they almost always do more harm than good when used over the long term.

If medicines are being prescribed for you, you should discuss this with your provider. It is not uncommon for people to have difficulty going off medications or alcohol. Also, stopping certain drugs suddenly *can* cause withdrawal symptoms. This leads us to take more medicine in order to alleviate them. We become caught in a vicious cycle of another order.

If you find yourself reluctant to talk to your prescriber for fear that he or she will stop your medication before you're ready, you may need some professional assistance. A counselor can help you to devise a more comfortable strategy for cutting back medications. You can then work out the details with your provider.

A typical first step is to change to a regular dosing schedule instead of just taking medication when you have pain. This can be done by tracking how much medicine you take in a typical week, then creating a regular weekly schedule that adds up to the same total. Every week after this, decrease the amount you take by 10 percent. Resist the urge to take a pill when you have more pain, and use mindful breathing, ice, heat, or stretching instead. Following these suggestions under the guidance of a professional, will allow most people to reduce and then eliminate their pain medication use.

If you find that you have become emotionally or physically dependent upon drugs or alcohol, joining a group program for substance problems such as Alcoholics Anonymous (AA) or Narcotics Anonymous (NA) can help.

FACING BIG DECISIONS

In the midst of chronic back pain, we may feel bad about not getting on with life. Decisions around career, relationships, having children, and education can easily get put on hold "until my back gets better." As you improve, however, you may become concerned about being able to handle the next steps. We can feel a bit like prisoners who, after a long time behind bars, grow frightened of living in the outside world.

Steven had graduated from college and was working in a frustrating job that didn't pay very well. He wanted to go back to school to prepare for a different career but couldn't decide what he wanted to do. He had suffered from lower back pain for years and was afraid that sitting in class for long periods would cause him terrible discomfort.

Steven put off the decision about school, waiting for his pain to go away. As he began to improve, however, he became unexpectedly anxious—he was now coming up against the old conflicts about choosing a career.

FEAR OF ABANDONING CONVENTIONAL TREATMENT

Another problem involves our long-term relationships with chiropractors, physical therapists, and other practitioners.

Harry had worked in construction for most of his life. He had come to accept back pain as part of the job. During the past couple of years, his pain was agonizing. He cut back on heavy lifting on the job and saw his chiropractor often.

Once he began to see that his problem was due to tension, Harry faced an unpleasant crossroads. He and the chiropractor had become friends over the years. The guy had always been there when he needed him, and Harry wanted to know that he would be there again, just in case this new way of dealing with the pain didn't work out.

Nonetheless, Harry realized that seeing his chiropractor was part of the problem—he treated Harry as though his spine were damaged. He had to try going without adjustments if he was ever going to believe that his back was okay. It took several months to summon the courage to tell his chiropractor that he was going to "take a break" from treatment.

Do you meet regularly with a back care professional who reinforces your apprehensions about your back? Are you concerned they may no longer be as dedicated to your well-being if you suspend treatment for a while?

RETURNING TO WORK

Disability payments can present another dilemma. You may want to return to work but be afraid that you won't be able to handle it. If you report to your disability examiner that you're okay, you'll lose your benefits and may have to return to work immediately. On the other hand, if you report that you're still disabled, you may not feel free to resume normal activities.

> *Cathy was a nurse who had been on disability for seven years because of back pain. She was miserable and very much wanted to return to work.*
>
> *She had made great strides but was afraid to do too much—not only out of fear of increased pain, but also out of fear that people would see her. She didn't want the neighbors to think that she was cheating the insurance company and feared that the company itself might check up on her.*
>
> *She was afraid that she was not yet able to handle real work but couldn't go further while she feared losing face and benefits. Nonetheless, when she finally took the plunge and told her employer that she was ready to work, something unmistakably changed. She began to be able to move and interact with people differently—no longer obligated to be in pain.*

If you are collecting disability or have an injury settlement pending, do concerns about earning a living or future medical costs make you hesitant to settle your case? Unfortunately, it has been repeatedly shown that this dilemma holds people back from getting better.

It is usually best to return to work, or at least light duty, as soon as possible. Many insurers now allow people to resume work part-time.

This is often a good compromise that can help overcome your concerns.

At this point, you have most of the tools that you will need to overcome back pain. Please remember, the process can require patience and perseverance. The next chapter provides specific instructions for developing an attitude of mindfulness.

CHAPTER 12

A GUIDE TO MINDFULNESS

THIS CHAPTER EXPLAINS:

- **How and why mindfulness techniques work**
- **How to use various mindfulness methods**
- **How to choose the most appropriate technique for you**

We have described the many ways that our natural emergency response system, the fight-or-flight reaction, all too often gets stuck in the *on* position. At many points in the book, we've advised you to use mindfulness to manage this problem, on the basis of fairly brief guidelines. We will now provide more in-depth directions to help you refine this widely applicable skill.

THE PERENNIAL PROBLEM

Stress reduction tactics of the ancients

Beginning thousands of years ago, many of the world's peoples felt a need to develop practices to calm the mind and body. Anthropologists theorize that early hunters discovered that they could remain still and alert for long periods by relaxing the fight-or-flight response. Some believe that the ancients also found that they could cure physical and emotional ills in this way. These eventually evolved into the meditation practices that are found in many world cultures today.

In recent years, scientists have extensively studied the effects of mindfulness techniques on both the body and the mind. A wide variety of them have been proven effective for treating stress-related problems. Perhaps the best-known studies in this area have been carried out by Dr. Herbert Benson, a cardiologist at Harvard Medical School, who called the effect of these the *relaxation response.* This is, in essence, the opposite of the fight-or-flight response. The relaxation response has been shown to boost the immune system, lower blood pressure, facilitate sleep, reduce tightness of muscles, slow brain waves, and relieve chronic pain.

Any method that brings about the relaxation response can interrupt the pain-fear-tension cycle. It can be used to cope effectively with the anxiety that usually accompanies expanding your range of activities, and it can help you tolerate pain without becoming overly stressed by it. Some of the techniques can also help you recognize and work with the underlying emotions that may be contributing to your tension and pain. All of them involve gently focusing your attention on something in the present moment with an accepting attitude. They all also involve letting go of the mind's usual preoccupations—the planning, worrying, judging, and problem solving that fill our days. The approaches share a *goal-less* quality—they don't necessarily produce relaxation or pain reduction each time you use them. Instead, you use them to relax the habit of fighting unpleasant sensations. As you practice mindfulness, you'll find that your fight-or-flight response calms down naturally.

As you become increasingly mindful, you may notice all sorts of emotions arising. As we discussed earlier, we don't try to change them but simply observe how the emotions feel in the body. When you do this for the first few times, you may feel as though you have opened a Pandora's box. Don't be alarmed. You will increasingly see that everything in life changes over time, and when we try too hard to control things, we just get aggravated. By using mindfulness in this way, you will feel stronger and less stressed.

For some people (especially if you've suffered through psychological trauma), mindfulness can bring up overwhelming thoughts and feelings. If this happens, it is best to use techniques that bring your attention to the world around you. For example, you might try walking meditation but turn your attention to your surroundings rather than the sensations in your body.

No one technique is effective for everyone. You can try several and see which ones come most easily to you. Certain methods are easier when you are relatively calm, while others will work better when you feel more restless.

BREATH MEDITATION

A simple procedure for focusing the mind

For some people, the word *meditation* conjures up exotic images of incense, gurus, and hippies. In fact, meditation is used by people of every description all over the world. Breath meditation in particular is one of the world's oldest and simplest ways to develop mindfulness. It is good to try first, because it will quickly help you to observe how restless your mind and body may be.

Try this experiment. Make a fist and squeeze hard. Hold it tightly for a few moments before reading further. Now notice what happened to your breathing? You probably either held your breath or found that it became shallower and more constricted.

Next try breathing deeply and slowly for a few moments. Make a fist again. Notice how it's different? Notice how your whole body is more relaxed? When we breathe completely, we tend not to become as tense.

We also tend to feel more, since we constrict our breathing somewhat when we hold back emotion. When a person is overwhelmed, others often suggest they "take a deep breath." In breath meditation, you use this same principle to your advantage.

To try breath meditation, you should set aside twenty minutes during which you will not be interrupted. (If you can manage it, research suggests that longer time periods, up to forty-five minutes, are even more effective.) If possible, choose a regular time of day. Use a timer so you don't have to watch the clock.

Find a comfortable, quiet, private place. Using a supportive chair, or a pillow on the floor, sit so that your spine is more or less straight. A straight spine will help you to feel alert. One way to find an upright posture is to imagine a string pulling you up from the top of your head toward the ceiling. Your hands can be folded or rest separately on your knees. (If you find sitting painful, you can begin practicing this lying down, though it can be difficult to stay awake in that position.)

Next close your eyes and begin to pay attention to the rising and falling sensations in your belly as you breathe in and out. As you inhale, you will notice that your belly rises slightly; as you exhale, you will notice your belly falls. Pay attention to the rising and falling sensations without trying to regulate your breath in any particular way. If these sensations are not apparent, try putting your hand gently on your stomach so you can feel them from the outside. Once the sensations are clear, you can lower your hands.

If you find that you scarcely notice your breathing, make a mental note of "rising" and "falling" as your belly moves. Simply repeat the words silently to yourself. This will help to anchor your attention.

Try to let your attention follow your breath, coming and going at its own pace. Some breaths will be long and deep, others short and shallow. At times the sensation of the breath may be very distinct, at other times faint. It may be rough or smooth. Your breath may come easily or may feel strained. There is no one *right* way for it to feel. All that you need to do is pay attention to it.

Before long, you will probably notice that your mind begins to wander. You may begin to notice other sensations in the body, be distracted by sounds, or lose yourself in thought or emotion. This is to be expected—it happens to everyone. As soon as you notice that your attention has wandered, however, bring it back to the rising and falling sensation. Many people soon notice that their mind is astoundingly busy and wanders off every few seconds. This is not a problem. Each time you notice that your mind has wandered off, simply bring your attention to the present. It will help your concentration to follow your breath closely, from beginning of inhalation, through the point of fullness, back down to the beginning of the next inhalation.

You may get sleepy or actually doze off. Most of the time we are pretty stressed, and as soon as we start to relax, we can easily drift into sleep. If you find it difficult to remain awake, try opening your eyes and letting your gaze focus softly on a spot several feet in front of you on the floor (or on the ceiling if you're lying down) as you continue to follow your breath.

One of the hardest parts of breath meditation is finding the best balance between effort and self-acceptance. If you don't try at all to bring your attention back to the sensations of the breath, you'll find yourself lost in thought the whole time. On the other hand, if you try *too* hard to focus on your breath, you'll become tense and agitated when your mind wanders. This is like puppy training—you tell the puppy to sit, but it wanders off over and over. Each time the puppy goes away, you gently bring it back. The trick is to do it all with an attitude of loving acceptance, understanding that, like a puppy, our minds are naturally very active.

When the time that you've set aside is over, gradually open your eyes. Don't get up right away. Take a few minutes to notice the room around you. Look at the colors and textures of the objects in the room. Notice the sounds and smells. Pay attention to the temperature and the feeling of the air on your body. Many people find that their environment becomes more vivid and that they notice more of what is happening around them.

At times, breath meditation may come easily. Your mind readily comes to rest "on the breath," and you feel comfortable. At other times, it may be quite difficult. You may find yourself lost in thought, irritable, or anxious. You feel restless, unfocused, or in pain. This is to be expected. All that you need to do is repeatedly bring your attention back to your breath, allowing your mind and body to go through their changes. Over time you will find that meditation gets easier.

While you are following your breath, painful sensations may appear. Allow them to come and go without trying to get rid of them. If they become strong, turn your attention to them for a while. Notice how sometimes the pain is sharp, sometimes dull. Sometimes it is intense, other times it is mild. It may move from place to place. You will eventually come to see that your pain is not a solid "thing." This is usually not obvious at first. Notice how it is really made up of a series of brief sensations strung together, the way a movie is composed of a series of still frames.

When you employ breath meditation, you notice more clearly the distinction between pain sensations per se and aversion responses to them. The pain sensations may be burning, aching, throbbing, or stabbing. When the sensations reach a certain intensity, we then notice our pain-distress thoughts: *Oh no, it's back. Damn—this isn't making it better, I hate this. Maybe I should get up and stretch,* and so on. You may notice signs of your fight-or-flight response accompanying these thoughts—a feeling of tension, breath shorter and shallower, heart rate increasing. As you notice these reactions, just again return your attention to your breath and observe how the pain sensations, and your responses to them, continue to change.

You can try to practice breath meditation daily for a period of several weeks in order to observe its positive effects. This can be tough if your life is busy or if some of the meditation sessions are uncomfortable. Nonetheless, most people who stick with it begin to appreciate its benefits.

QUESTIONS ABOUT BREATH MEDITATION

I notice that my belly doesn't move at all when I breathe. Am I doing something wrong? If you find that your belly doesn't move when breathing, it is likely that your breath is confined to your chest. If you discover this, you may find the following to be of use: Lie down and place one hand on your chest and the other on your belly. Now imagine each time that you breathe in, a balloon begins to fill inside your belly. Each time you breathe out, imagine the balloon shrinking. Soon you'll notice that your belly rises and falls more with each breath and your chest moves less. Most people find that breathing this way soon feels very natural and easy. This style of breathing tends to be more calming than chest breathing.

When I sit quietly, my pain seems to get worse. Is this normal? When we've been in pain for a long time, we naturally try to find ways to distract ourselves. When you first slow down and turn your attention to your breath, you can be alarmed by how intense the pain sensations are. This does not mean that you're doing anything wrong or that you're making your pain worse. In fact, research suggests that distraction ultimately may make pain worse. You will find that accepting the pain sensations will make them more tolerable and less distressing.

My mind is incredibly active. I'm always lost in thought. Does this mean there's something wrong with me? Most people are alarmed to find just how busy their minds are when they first try breath meditation. In our culture we are bombarded with stimulation—both from busy lives and from the intense images in the media. Our ancestors living in nature would have probably been totally overwhelmed by the stimulation we experience during an ordinary trip to the mall. Try to be patient with yourself. If you practice breath meditation regularly, you'll eventually find that it becomes a bit easier, and your mind will become more relaxed. If you find that your mind is terribly restless, however, you may find it easier to use one of the other methods we will discuss shortly.

When I sit quietly I get very anxious. Frightening thoughts and feelings come into my mind. Should I keep trying? When we begin to slow down and sit quietly, we notice thoughts and feelings that we are usually distracted from. For some people, especially those who have suffered psychological trauma from abuse or being exposed to violence, these can include unhappy memories. If you feel emotionally overwhelmed, stop for now and try walking meditation.

I've done breath meditation for a couple of weeks, but I still feel distracted a lot. Does this mean it's not working? Many people imagine, from things they've heard, that their minds should become blank while meditating. Although it is true that some people develop states of completely engrossing concentration, this takes a great deal of time and isn't our goal here. A meditation teacher once said, "If you have a mind, it is going to wander." There will always be some days in which you're more distracted. You are practicing accepting all of the thoughts, sensations, and emotions that arise, including the distractions.

WORD MEDITATION

Adding meaning to mindfulness

There are several variations on simple breath meditation that some people find come more naturally to them. One type involves the use of *mantras*—words or phrases repeated silently in the mind with each breath. Mantras can be useful both for helping the mind to focus and for evoking calming, comforting feelings.

Here is an area where your particular personality, religion, and cultural background matter. If you are nonreligious, you can simply use the words *rising* and *falling* to help your mind to focus. You might find it helpful to use other words or phrases that you associate with feeling safe or calm. Good candidates, some of which have been used in research on the relaxation response, include *one, relax, peace, let it be,* or *love.* You simply repeat the word or phrase silently with each breath. Most people find it works best to repeat it each time they exhale.

If you are religious, using a word or short phrase from a prayer may help you let go of fears and concerns. Many people like to repeat phrases such as *Our Father who art in heaven, The Lord is my shepherd, Shalom,* or others from their background that evoke feelings of peace.

Studies have shown that people with religious conviction have better odds of getting over illness. Faith can help us to accept what is happening by enabling us to put our trust in something larger than ourselves. This allows us to relax our need for control, relax our fight against pain, and develop an accepting attitude.

If you are still doubtful of the potential impact of practices derived from religion upon a medical condition, it might interest you to know that research conducted at Duke University suggested that participating in religious services is associated with a significant increase in length of life. The study drew on a large sample of four thousand individuals and found that going to services was as beneficial to longevity as not smoking.

As with simple breath meditation, you will probably find your mind wandering when you use your word or phrase. The instructions here are exactly the same—as soon as you notice that your mind has strayed, gently bring it back. Remember, you're not trying to fight with your mind and force it to concentrate.

SELF-SUGGESTION

A variation of word meditation involves what is called *self-suggestion.* Once you've been meditating for a while, and your mind quiets down, you may wish to try it. Silently repeat to yourself a series of phrases that address whatever part of the process you've been having difficulty with. For example, if you find yourself generally trying too hard to control your pain, you might think, *May I no longer fear pain, May I come to accept things the way they are.* You simply repeat these phrases over and over for several minutes. The ideas can be more general as well, such as *May I be happy. May I be peaceful. May I be free from suffering.* They can also be directed at others, such as *May my family be happy. May my family be free from suffering.* You may find that your feelings begin to "respond" to the words you repeat.

QUESTIONS ABOUT WORD MEDITATION

When I try word meditation, I find myself changing my word a lot, trying to find the one that works best. Is this a good idea? For most people, it is best to settle on a word or phrase and stay with it for a period of days or weeks. Otherwise you can become preoccupied with finding the "best" word. Once you have practiced for a while, you can experiment with another word.

I've been pretty discouraged about my pain. Even though I repeat a positive phrase, I keep thinking angry, negative thoughts. What should I do? We all feel a mix of positive and negative feelings much of the time. When we begin to emphasize the positive, we often find opposite feelings appearing. While these negative feelings may not seem admirable, they're perfectly normal. There's no need to fight with your mind.

WALKING MEDITATION

Mindfulness in motion

For some people, methods that require remaining still are too confining. If this is true for you, try walking meditation. Most people find that they can do this no matter what mood they may be in.

Begin by finding an area, indoors or out, where you can comfortably walk back and forth, about twenty steps in each direction. Take a few moments at first to close your eyes, and notice your breathing and the sensations throughout your body. Notice the sensations of your weight on the soles of your feet as you stand on the ground. Begin to walk slowly, paying attention to the sensations of your legs moving and of your feet touching the ground. Try to follow the sensations involved in each step. Notice your foot lifting off the ground, moving forward, and making contact again. See how your weight shifts from left to right. The idea is to use the sensations of walking as a focus of your attention.

When you get to the other end of the path on which you are walking, pause for a moment, continuing to feel the sensations in your body. Then turn slowly and head back to your starting point. Continue walking slowly, back and forth. As with breath meditation, continue for at least twenty minutes each time.

You will probably find your mind wandering again. When this happens simply come back to noticing the sensations of walking.

Here, too, you may want to repeat words to help you stay focused. If you feel distracted, try walking very slowly. Lift one foot gradually and say silently, *Lifting.* Next move it forward, repeating, *Forward.* Finally place the foot down and say, *Placing.* Repeat these words in your mind as you lift each foot, bring it forward, and place it down. During each step, try to pay attention to the sensations in your legs and feet. While walking slowly and attentively may feel peculiar at first, you will soon notice that it is very effective.

The idea here isn't to *walk* in a particular way—walking meditation isn't designed for physical exercise. After doing this for a number of days, you'll increasingly notice that walking around the house, doing errands, or going for a stroll are all opportunities to practice.

While some people think of meditation as eccentric, a number of HMOs (health maintenance organizations), known for their strict attention to the bottom-line effectiveness of treatments, have turned to the use of mindfulness to assist their patients. Plan members referred for these nontraditional treatments include those suffering from high blood pressure, depression, anxiety, and various pain conditions that have been shown to respond to mindfulness and relaxation states in numerous studies.

Almost any situation can provide opportunities to employ mindfulness. Mindfulness is sometimes also described as "opening to God" or "receiving the Holy Spirit." Prayer, chanting, singing hymns, yoga, and other practices can be used to cultivate it. If you have interest in any of these, by all means use them.

In the next chapter we will tackle the physical dimension of back pain by guiding you through a systematic program to develop strength, flexibility, and confidence in the strength in your back.

CHAPTER 13

A GUIDE TO REGAINING FITNESS

THIS CHAPTER EXPLAINS:

- Why formal physical exercise is an important part of the Back Sense program
- How to get permission for exercise from your doctor
- General principles for exercise
- Specific ways to increase your strength, flexibility, and endurance

EXERCISE NOW!

Why an exercise program is especially important

If you are like most people, you began limiting your movements in reaction to your pain. Unhappily, because the back is central to almost everything we do, this means abandoning a wide range of activity. Avoiding movement that we associate with our pain tightens our muscles; reduces our strength, endurance, and range of motion; and keeps us fearful.

Chapter 8 started you on the process of resuming life. You began with things that were both enjoyable and not too frightening to resume. Gradually you increased the intensity and duration of the activities, moving toward the goal of behaving like somebody who never had back trouble in the first place. While this steady, step-by-step return is enough to break the back pain cycle for some people, most sufferers also benefit from a systematic exercise program.

While many back pain programs and books include exercises for strengthening, stretching, or protecting the back, it is critical to realize that our main purpose is entirely different. The exercises we outline are *not* presented as necessary to protect your "weak" back or to allow your "damaged" back to heal. They are designed instead to build your confidence and to help you see that your back is actually quite rugged. Once you prove to yourself that you can lift, bend, and exert yourself vigorously, you will no longer need to fear playing sports or lifting a bag of groceries.

Being strong and flexible also reduces the chances of experiencing the minor injuries that can cause acute (short-lived) back pain. In addition, exercise provides relief from stress and tension.

As we've discussed, an overwhelming number of well-designed research studies now very clearly confirm that an aggressive restoration of full functioning is the quickest way to leave pain and disability behind.

PERMISSION TO MOVE FREELY

Getting approval from your doctor to go forward

Before beginning, it is important to check with your physician to see if there are any exercise restrictions that you need to follow because of your age or particular medical problems. Some people will need an exercise stress test to determine the safe amount of exercise for them.

Medical situations that may require a modified program include osteoporosis, diabetes, high blood pressure, a smoking history, high cholesterol, or an immediate family member who developed heart disease before age fifty-five. In addition, the following symptoms may require further diagnostic testing and/or modification of your exercise program: pain or discomfort in the chest that appears to be from the heart; shortness of breath upon mild exertion or when lying down or trying to sleep; dizziness or passing out; ankle swelling; heart palpitations or a heart murmur; or leg pain from poor blood circulation. Medications that you are taking should also be reviewed with your physician.

By stressing certain points, you can make it easier for your health practitioner to let you progress with exercise. Emphasize to him or her that you are looking only to rule out serious medical problems. Tell your practitioner that you want to exercise and are aware that this may cause a temporary increase in your back pain. You may want to ask, "If I didn't have a back problem, would there be any limitations on my starting an exercise program?"

GENERAL GUIDELINES FOR EXERCISE

How to plan a safe and effective program

There are certain principles you should keep in mind as you begin regular exercise:

1. Understand from the beginning that you need to set aside some time for exercise. Twenty to forty-five minutes per session, at least three times a week, is needed. When you are starting the program, it is good to do the same exercises every day, so you can begin to have the experience of the pain varying—while your level of physical activity remains the same.

2. Understand that getting into shape will take a while if you have been limiting your movement and have become decondi-

tioned. Depending on your present state of fitness and other factors, you may need to begin with lighter weights and more gradual stretching. Also, there may be large variations in how quickly "normal" condition is reached. It is important to set targets that are attainable and realistic.

We recommend setting both short-term goals (for the week) and long-term goals (for the next two months). You can increase what you are doing every three sessions or at minimum once a week. Six to eight weeks will usually allow most people to become fit enough for normal day-to-day functioning, though it may not be enough time to allow for return to very physically demanding jobs or atheletic competition. We recommend at least another three months of continued stretching, strength, and endurance training after completing the exercise sequence. The general health benefits of exercise cannot be overstated. Many people find that they continue this routine indefinitely after they have had a taste of being in shape.

3. Some degree of pain and fatigue cannot be avoided during reconditioning. As we have stated throughout this book, adopting an accepting attitude toward pain is essential. In the first few weeks of an exercise program, it is completely normal to experience some increase in pain. Try not to worry too much. You are encountering both the pain of a sedentary person getting into condition and the increased pain that results from the anxiety and tension of the chronic pain syndrome.

People sometimes, understandably, confuse the "good" pain that temporarily results from using long-neglected muscles with the pain of their "bad back." Use mindfulness, application of a hot or cold pack, or occasional nonprescription pain relievers (see appendix 2) to manage discomfort. Remember, though, that the goal of the exercise program is not to eliminate your pain.

It is also important to remember, especially for those who may have never been in good physical condition, that breathing hard, feeling your heart beat quickly, and sweating are all normal parts of exercise. While these sensations may feel uncomfortable at first, you will probably come to enjoy them.

4. Use measurements and goals to record your progress, rather than your own sense of how hard you are pushing or how you are coming along. Using a personal feeling of fatigue or stretch to measure changes in endurance or flexibility often leads to no real gains. People can feel they are doing everything that can be done yet remain inflexible and weak. This can be discouraging. On the other hand, keeping a written record of your progress is motivating. We recommend that you use the simple charts that are included here.

5. There is no need to become overly compulsive about exercise. Once they begin to feel better, some people become upset about missing a day at the gym, fearing that their back will become weak again and they will backslide. Please remember, the primary purpose of this exercise is to gain confidence. Missing a day here and there is nothing to be concerned about.

FLEXIBILITY TRAINING

Stretching and relaxing your muscles

There are three complementary types of exercise that can help you revitalize your back. The first, *flexibility training,* simply involves *stretching.* It serves to lengthen and relax muscles so as to increase their range of motion as well as reduce the pain and soreness associated with tightness. Almost everyone with long-standing back pain develops a problem with flexibility. This usually affects forward and backward bending the most.

All of the following stretches are best performed at least three times a week. They can be done several times a day if you desire. Stretching should be done gradually and slowly in a warm place. It is also good to warm up by walking briskly prior to stretching, recalling how your body felt before you had problems with back pain.

A good rule of thumb during a stretch is to let gravity do the work. Don't try to force your muscles to stretch by bouncing. Use slow, relaxed breathing and allow your muscles to gently relax on their own. It is very common for people to hold their breath in anticipation of pain, often without realizing it, and this adds to tightness. Imagine that you are directing your breath to ease the tension. With each breath you will notice your body moving slightly farther. A stretch should be held for at least thirty seconds to be most effective. Pay attention to your breathing, body sensations, thoughts, and feelings.

You may find worries about injury come back as you stretch, and you may experience various emotions. Stretching often releases held-in feelings.

To measure your progress, tape a piece of poster board to a wall and mark how far your fingertips reach during the forward, backward (easier to mark with a helper), left side, and right side stretches. This will help you to measure your increased flexibility. You can also see changes in your range of motion by watching yourself stretch in a mirror.

We have included *rough estimates* of what you might expect your increase in reach to be for each exercise. Remember, these are only approximations. Making faster or slower progress is fine, as long as you are steadily increasing your flexibility.

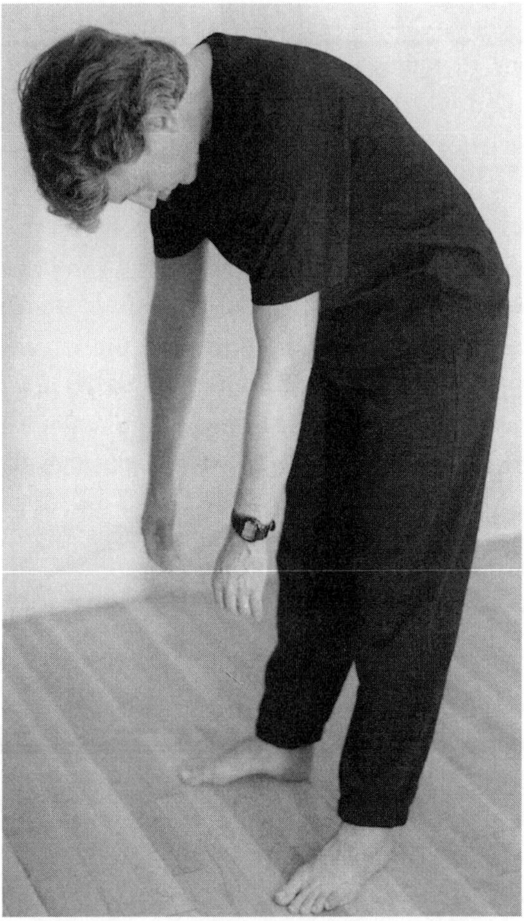

FORWARD STRETCH:

(Two-inch increase per week) Start by standing with your feet about six inches apart and your knees straight. Look down and gradually allow your head to droop forward. Once you feel a stretch in the back of your neck, slowly begin to reach down with your hands toward the ground. Feel the tightness in your legs and back while you gently breathe into the stretch. Allow yourself to hang, with gravity gradually lengthening your muscles. After hanging for as long as you are comfortable, mark your position on the wall and slowly roll back up, starting at the base of your spine, until you are vertical again. Make sure to breathe during the whole process.

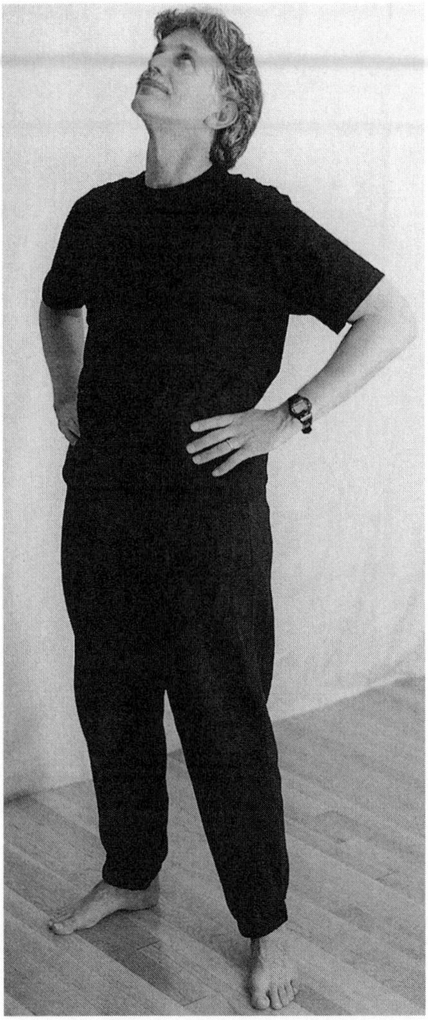

BACKWARD STRETCH:

(One-half-inch increase per week) Start from the same posture as the forward stretch. Put your hands on your hips and gently start to move your whole spine backward while looking up at the ceiling. Again, let gravity do the stretching, while you breathe slowly and deeply. When you are at your maximum stretch, you can put your hands down and behind you to measure your progress on the wall. Slowly return to vertical.

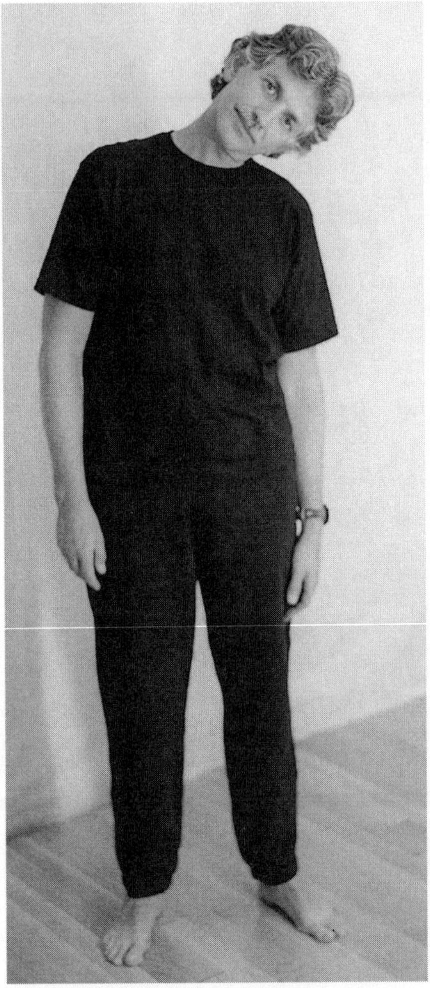

SIDE STRETCHES:

(One-inch increase per week) Again, begin by standing up straight. Next allow your head to droop to the left. Once you feel a stretch in your neck, gently slide your left hand down your leg toward the floor, feeling the stretch on your right side, breathing, and letting yourself hang. Mark your position on the wall and slowly roll back up, starting with your waist until you are vertical. Repeat on the other side.

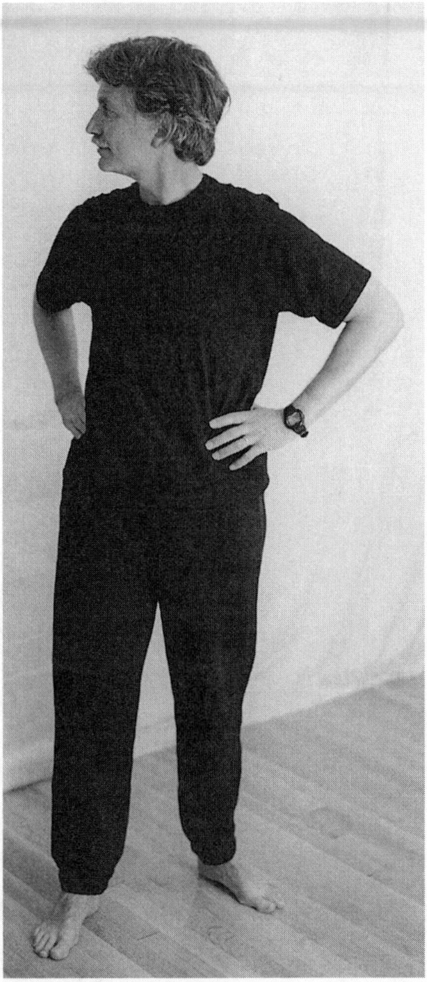

SIDE ROTATIONS:

Keeping your feet planted, put your hands on your hips and gently rotate your upper body as far as you can go without straining. This stretch is harder to measure, but if you start in the same position every time, you can mentally mark a spot on the wall that you can see when you are most rotated. Try to move this spot farther each time you do this stretch. Repeat, rotating the other way.

Many people find stretching makes them feel calmer as well as relieving sensations of muscle tightness. If it works well for you, try the following positions. They are all done on the floor, using a carpet or mat for cushioning:

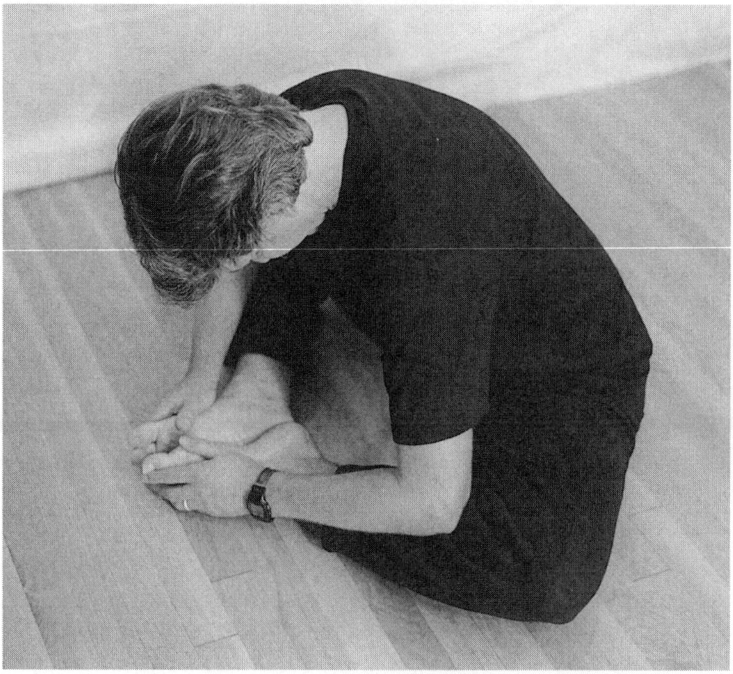

FEET TOGETHER FORWARD STRETCH:

With your knees bent, touch the soles of your feet together in front of you. Now gently lean forward, allowing your head to droop, and breathe. Next, gradually turn your torso so that your chest is over your left knee, let yourself hang, and again breathe into the tightness. Next, gradually face forward, and continue turning until your chest is over your right knee. Hang, hold this posture, and breathe, then return to facing forward.

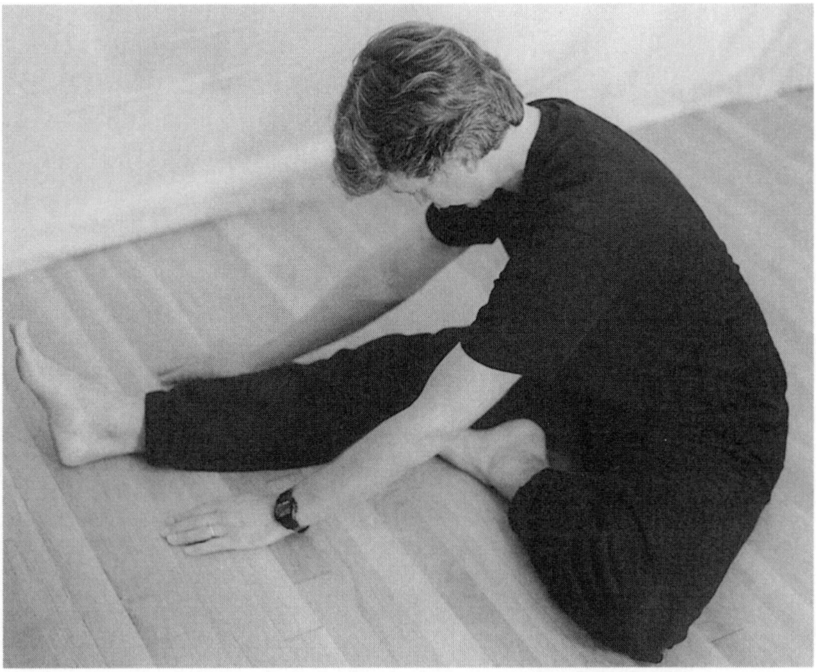

HAMSTRING STRETCH:

Place your right leg straight out in front of you and bend your left leg so that the sole of your left foot touches the inside of your right leg. Gently lean forward, allowing your head to droop, and breathe into wherever you feel tightness. Next, reverse the position of your legs, placing your left leg straight in front, bending your right leg so that the sole of your right foot touches the inside of your left leg. Again gently lean forward and breathe into the stretch.

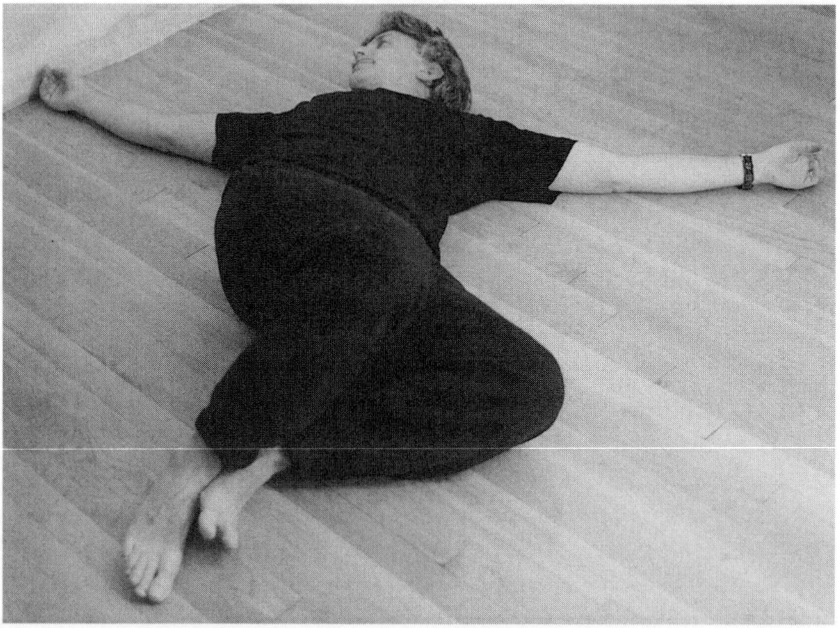

BACK ROTATION:

Lie on your back and gently bring your knees to your chest, allowing your feet to come off the floor. Hold your knees with your arms and breathe into any tightness you feel. Next, allow your arms to rest on the floor, sticking straight out from your body. Keeping your knees bent, gradually allow them to fall toward your left side, while your shoulders remain against the floor. Breathe in this position. Next, bring your knees up to the starting position near your chest, and allow them to cross over to your right side, again keeping your shoulders on the floor. Breathe again. Finish with your knees against your chest, holding them again with your arms.

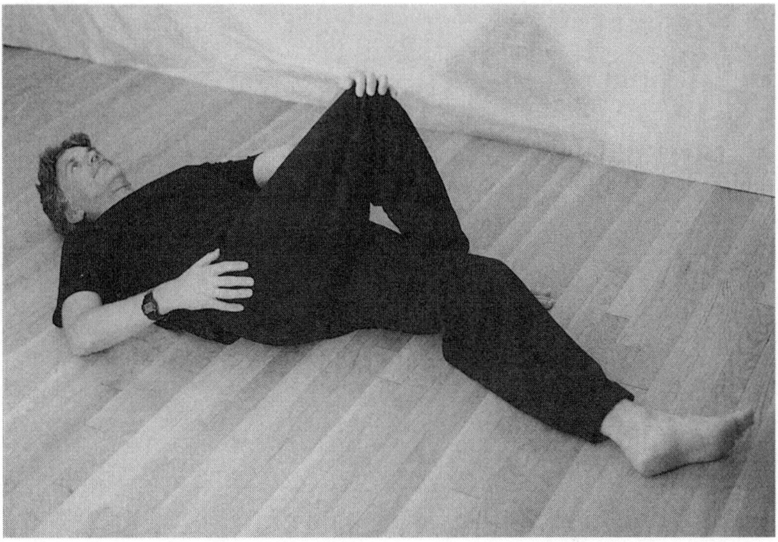

PYRIFORMIS STRETCH:

Lie on your back, with your right knee bent, pointing up, and your left leg flat on the floor. Place the sole of your right foot on floor, on the outside of your left thigh. Keeping your hips on the floor, gently pull your right knee left and downward until you feel a stretch deep in your buttocks. Breathe slowly and deeply while continuing this gentle pull. Next, reverse the position of your legs and gently pull your left leg downward, toward the right, again breathing slowly.

These stretches address most major muscle groups connected with back pain. If they do not seem to stretch a muscle that you find particularly tight or painful, you can invent your own stretch. Simply place yourself in the position that has been sensitive and stretch just to the first point of discomfort. Adopting the position you may have most dreaded can provide a real confidence boost.

STRENGTH TRAINING

Developing strong muscles that you aren't afraid to use

The second type of exercise, *strength training,* is designed to reverse the gradual weakening of muscles that occurs as a result of too much rest and constricted movement. Even if you have kept up with normal life, you probably protect or guard your back to some extent, which causes weakness. Strength training often employs weights to provide resistance to the action of muscles and make them work harder. Two factors influence the effects it has on a muscle: *intensity* (the amount of resistance and speed of movement) and *duration* (the length of time during which exercises are done). Strengthening should be done at least three times a week, although it is ideal to do it daily. Strengthening many muscles is optimal, but it is most important to exercise the lifting muscles and back extension muscles (the muscles that allow us to bend backward), as we are usually most afraid to use these normally when we have back pain.

To measure your progress, photocopy the strength training logs provided here to keep track of both the weight you use and the number of repetitions of the exercises. You can use dumbbells or a simple plastic crate filled with anything that adds weight, such as cans of food or books. The crate can easily be weighed with a bathroom scale. If you find the suggested weights too easy, they may be slowly increased. It is not so important what weight you start at, but you should see measurable increases every week. It is also important to watch your pulse so that you know how your heart is responding to this exercise (see following section on endurance training).

GUIDELINES FOR WEIGHT LIFTING

GENDER AND HEIGHT	STARTING WEIGHT	WEEKLY INCREASE	FINAL GOAL
Females under 5' 4"	10 lbs.	2 lbs.	26 lbs.
Females 5' 4" or over	15 lbs.	2 lbs.	31 lbs.
Males under 5' 8"	15 lbs.	2 lbs.	31 lbs.
Males 5' 8" or over	20 lbs.	2 lbs.	36 lbs.

Note: If you are over fifty-five years old, decrease the starting and final weight goals by 5 lbs. each.

You should start with five repetitions for the first week and increase by two each week until you reach fifteen repetitions. This will get you to your final goal in six weeks.

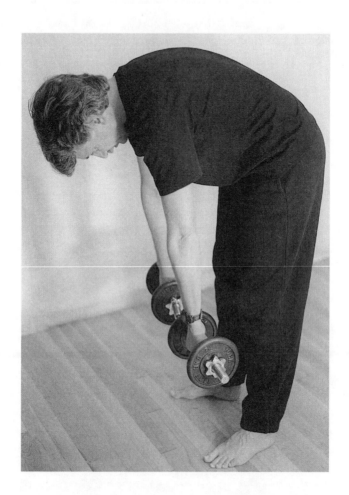

FLOOR-TO-WAIST LIFT:

Lift the crate or dumbbells from the floor to waist height (it can be placed on a table). It is best to lift as a child would, without thinking about technique. Contrary to what you may have heard, there is *no reason* to lift using only your legs. You may in fact neglect important muscles if you always try to keep your back rigid. Remember to breathe while you are exercising, as this will help to keep your muscles relaxed.

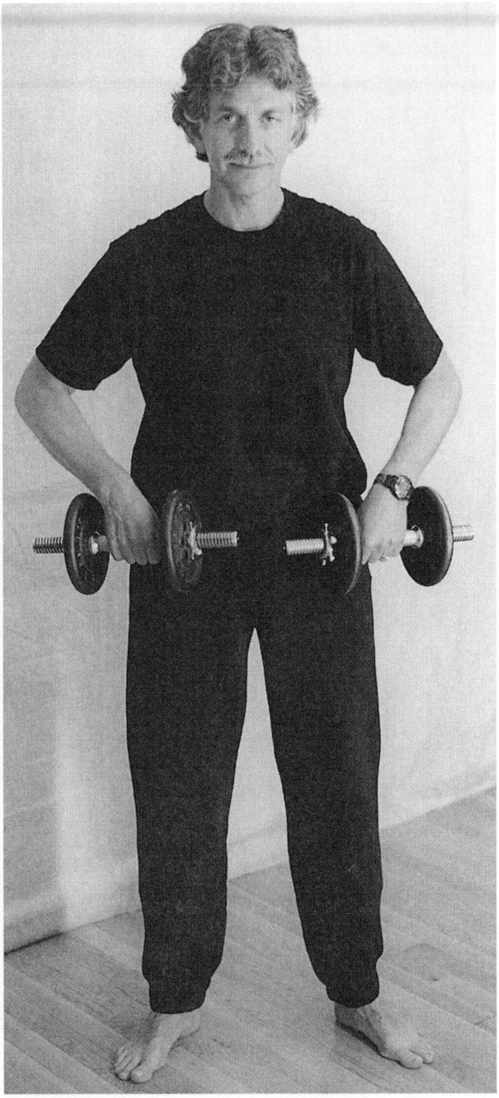

WAIST-TO-CHEST LIFT:

Lift the crate from waist height to shoulder height (you can lift the crate from a table to a high shelf or bureau). Again, don't forget to breathe.

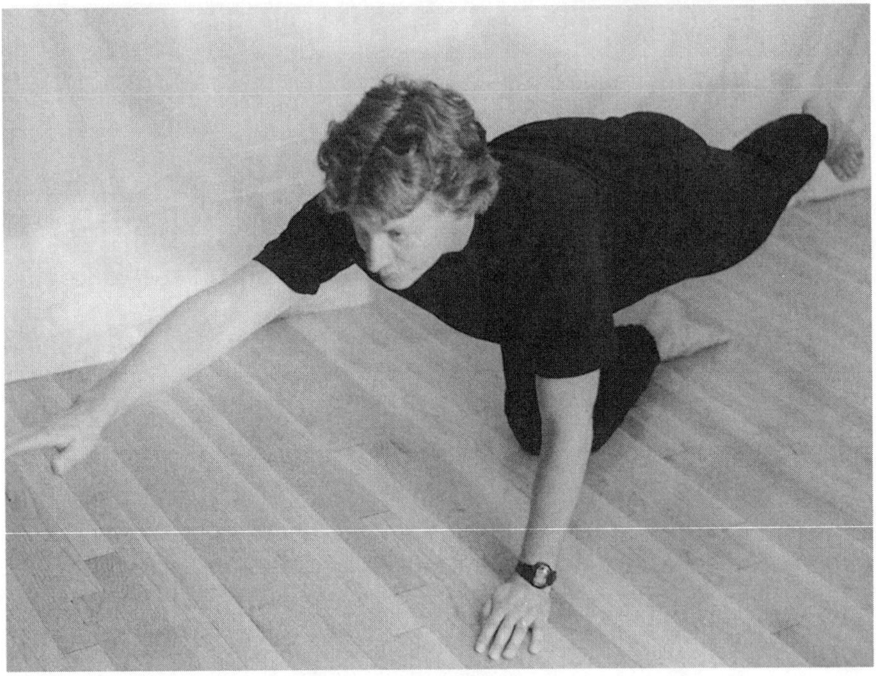

BACK EXTENSION:

Get on the floor on your hands and knees. Gently lift your left leg, point it out straight back, and hold it there. Now raise your right arm and point it out straight ahead. Hold this position for a slow count of five, then relax. Repeat with the right leg and the left arm extended. If you have difficulty with this, you can leave your hands on the ground and just point your leg backward. Repeat this exercise five times initially. Each week, increase your repetitions by two and your hold time by two seconds, until you reach a goal of fifteen repetitions of ten-second holds.

STRENGTH TRAINING LOG—
FLOOR-TO-WAIST LIFT

Use this table to record the weight you use with an *X*, referring to the column at the left. Each column should be used for one session. Fill in the date of each session at the bottom.

POUNDS LIFTED

40																			
39																			
38																			
37																			
36																			
35																			
34																			
33																			
32																			
31																			
30																			
29																			
28																			
27																			
26																			
25																			
24																			
23																			
22																			
21																			
20																			
19																			
18																			
17																			
16																			
15																			
14																			
13																			
12																			
11																			
10																			
Date																			

STRENGTH TRAINING LOG—WAIST-TO-CHEST LIFT

Use this table to record the weight you use with an *X*, referring to the column at the left. Each column should be used for one session. Fill in the date of each session at the bottom.

POUNDS LIFTED

40																			
39																			
38																			
37																			
36																			
35																			
34																			
33																			
32																			
31																			
30																			
29																			
28																			
27																			
26																			
25																			
24																			
23																			
22																			
21																			
20																			
19																			
18																			
17																			
16																			
15																			
14																			
13																			
12																			
11																			
10																			
Date																			

ENDURANCE TRAINING

For confidence, health, and managing stress

The third type of exercise, *endurance training,* is also often called *aerobics.* The term *aerobics* is sometimes misunderstood as referring to specific *kinds* of exercises, such as "step aerobics." It actually means only that muscles are gradually improving the efficiency with which they use oxygen. This is how the body increases its ability to endure exertion. An overwhelming body of scientific research now indicates that aerobic exercise is vital to overall health, including heart, lung, and immune system functioning. It has been proven to lower overall stress and tension while combating anxiety and depression. Aerobic fitness does *not* require participation in organized groups like aerobics classes. It does require that you regularly (at least three times a week) participate in some activity that raises your pulse and breathing rate significantly. This usually involves breaking a sweat.

Some of the things that can provide a good aerobic workout, using minimal equipment, are biking, brisk walking, jogging, stair climbing, fast swimming, singles tennis, racquetball, and hiking. The simplest form of endurance training is brisk walking. This is very safe and available to anyone without equipment. If the weather is bad, many people have malls or other indoor spaces available to them.

It is obviously easiest to stick with a routine you enjoy. This might mean doing it in a park or while listening to music. Motorized treadmills have been shown to have a higher rate of continued use than other exercise equipment, possibly because all you have to do is set the pace and keep up with the machine. The mindfulness techniques we described in the last chapter can be combined with aerobic exercise, for those who have limited time.

To measure your progress, you can photocopy the endurance training log provided here to keep tabs on both intensity and duration. The *intensity* of aerobic exercise is best tracked using your pulse rate.

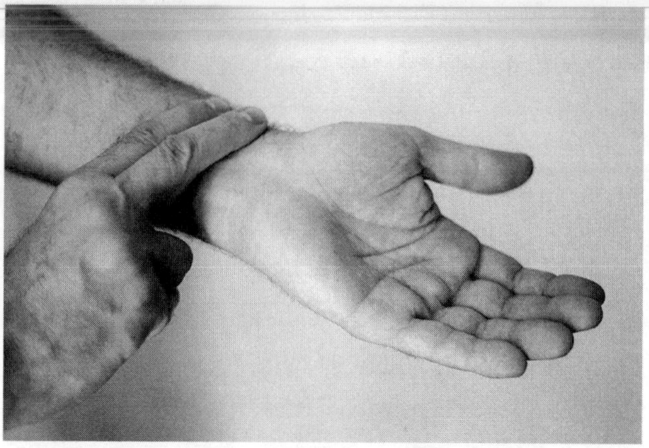

TAKING YOUR PULSE:
Put your left hand out, palm up. Find your pulse by using the tips of the first and second fingers of your right hand to press down firmly on the left side of the wrist, just below where the hand meets the wrist.

Estimate your pulse rate (per minute) by taking it for fifteen seconds and multiplying by four. The pulse rate you are shooting for is known as your *target heart rate.* The *duration* of exercise should be measured in minutes.

Practice finding your pulse before exercise, as it can get a little more difficult when you are moving. If you have trouble, many sporting supply stores sell devices that take your pulse automatically.

Here are the target heart rate goals for most people:

AGE	TARGET HEART RATE ZONE
25	136–156
30	133–152
35	129–148
40	126–144
45	122–140
50	119–136
55	115–132
60	112–128
65	108–124
70	105–120

These rates are guidelines. If you are new to exercise, you should start with a lower goal. You may find that your heart rate will vary by 10 percent above or below your goal in a typical session. Your physician can tell you if these target heart rates are appropriate for you.

Start with five minutes of exercise that brings your pulse to your target heart rate. Each week add two minutes. This will bring you to twenty minutes in about seven weeks. Twenty minutes is a good goal and should condition your heart and lungs, while providing an opportunity for stress reduction.

If you experience chest pain, excessive shortness of breath (breathing hard during exercise is normal) light-headedness, or any other unusual symptoms, you should stop the exercise program and see your physician. Also, be aware that certain blood pressure medicines prevent your heart rate from rising normally during exercise. This means you can't use the heart rate guidelines we provide. Your physician can help design a safe exercise program.

RETURNING TO FITNESS

You can go as far as you wish

The program we have outlined here will be effective if followed, but it is conservative. The fitness goals we have suggested are sufficient to help you to feel okay about performing most daily activities within approximately two months. If you would like a faster or more aggressive program, you may wish to seek additional guidance. Most people are able to develop considerably greater strength and endurance if they wish to.

If you want to develop your physical capacities further, or find that you are having trouble exercising on your own, we recommend going to a gym or health club. Most of these can provide a structure for working out if you have never been very physically industrious.

If you have worked out prior to your problem with back pain, you can return to any balanced exercise program that served you well. Remember, good programs include a combination of flexibility, strength, and endurance training. Just follow your doctor's advice about resuming exercise gradually if you have been sedentary for a long time.

ENDURANCE LOG

Use this table to record the number of minutes you exercise with an *X*, referring to the column at the left. Each column should be used for one session. Fill in the date of each session at the bottom of the column. Record your target heart rate in the row labeled H.R.

MINUTES OF EXERCISE

30																			
29																			
28																			
27																			
26																			
25																			
24																			
23																			
22																			
21																			
20																			
19																			
18																			
17																			
16																			
15																			
14																			
13																			
12																			
11																			
10																			
9																			
8																			
7																			
6																			
5																			
H.R.																			
Date																			

CHAPTER 14

FINAL THOUGHTS

ADVICE FROM THE OTHER SHORE

What people who have recovered recommend

We asked patients who had been through the program and recovered to tell us, "Based on your experience, what are the most important things for people with chronic back pain to know?" While each person's list is a little different, here is their collective advice:

- Remind yourself over and over about the true cause of your pain. Tell yourself, *My back is okay, my muscles are tense.* It can take a while for this to sink in.

- Don't buy every diagnosis or piece of advice you are given. Many physicians, chiropractors, and other professionals just don't understand what really causes the pain.

- Get a good evaluation from a doctor who understands what really causes back pain, so that you can move ahead.

- Don't waste your money on gadgets.

- Pay close attention to see if your back pain ever gets better and worse or changes location. It means there's a good chance it's caused by stress.

- If you've had other stress-related problems, your back pain is probably another one.

- Don't panic if you have a flare-up. Don't worry about what you've done to yourself physically.

- Keep an eye on your other problems in life besides back pain.

- Resolve to live normally. Don't let the pain stop you. Concentrate on getting your life back.

- Exercise.

- Try meditation or yoga. Learn how to accept the pain and to let go of fear and stress.

- If you develop other symptoms, don't despair. You're not falling apart. It simply means that tension is in fact the problem, and it's affecting another part of your body.

- Keep trying. Don't be too discouraged if the pain is intense, lasts for a long time, or comes back. You'll learn to handle it better each time it happens.

- Learn to see your pain as a harmless barometer of stress.

- Get help from people who understand how this works if you get stuck.

LOOKING FORWARD

What to expect in the future

Each part of the Back Sense program works with the other parts. The work you do expanding activities helps you to resolve some of the emotional parts of the problem, while the work you do in addressing emotions reduces your stress and makes it easier to expand your activity. Mindfulness and exercise both make it easier to handle troublesome emotions and to live a more normal life.

The exact pattern of recuperation is different for everyone. For some, increasingly long periods of reduced pain occur right away, and the pain rarely resurfaces. For others, the process of improvement is slower and requires greater patience. This is especially likely if the problem has existed for a long time and muscles are seriously deconditioned.

Back pain sometimes recurs after a person has felt significantly better. Many people feel devastated the first time this happens. They think, *I thought I had overcome this. Now I've reinjured myself and I'm right back where I started.* This can start the whole pain cycle going again. Don't get alarmed if your pain returns. New pain episodes typically last for only a few days if you continue normal behavior and pay attention to the stressors that may have caused them. It is vital to realize that feeling pain again does not mean you are stuck back at the beginning. You have learned to understand the cause of the pain and how to deal with it.

APPENDIX 1

MEDICAL DIAGNOSIS OF BACK PAIN

THE HEALTH HISTORY

Though people often think that the hands-on exam and diagnostic tests are the most important parts of a back pain–related doctor's appointment, physicians usually learn more from taking a careful history. Your doctor should ask you about other illnesses, how the pain started, whether the pain is getting gradually better or worse, other symptoms you might have that could indicate more serious causes of the back pain, what specific factors make the pain better or worse, and what diagnostic tests have already been performed.

As age increases (particularly over fifty), one needs to be much more alert to the possibility of serious medical causes of back pain. For this reason, more diagnostic testing is often performed with older patients. It is important to remember, however, that even among older people, most back pain is caused by muscle tension.

Practitioners will want to know how the pain started. You may have been lifting, or a minor twist or pull made you feel a "pop" in your back, and the pain gradually worsened over the next few days. Both of these usually suggest a muscular problem. You may also have been in a motor vehicle accident, either with or without an injury. Although pain following accidents is often muscle related, here, too, physicians are more likely to order X-rays or a bone scan to make sure there is not a fracture. Often pain comes on gradually, without any specific incident. This tends to increase the doctor's attention to the possibility of other diagnoses. Again, however, most of the time this is muscular back pain.

The length of time that your pain has lasted is important. Most *acute* episodes of back pain get better on their own. It is common for physicians to do little testing if the pain has lasted for less than a month and there are no other significant findings in the exam or health history.

If the pain lasts for more than a month, further testing may be conducted, particularly if the pain is getting steadily worse. On the other hand, pain that lasts more than a year, or gets better and worse, is almost always muscular. Most other problems would have gotten either better or worse. Some types of arthritis may also cause long-lasting back pain, but this is easy to identify, since pain from arthritis will usually respond quite well to medications, while pain from muscles generally does not.

Determining the specific location of the pain is often useful since, for example, pain located more in the leg than in the back can occasionally indicate a disk problem. This can be quite misleading, however, as tightness of muscles also commonly causes leg pain (sciatica). When muscles in the buttocks area tighten, they can cause pressure or a temporary decrease in blood flow to the nerves in our legs. This can produce pain or numbness down your leg, though it doesn't cause any damage to the nerves. While sciatica is often thought by both doctors and average people to be associated with a pinched nerve in the back, it is much more commonly caused by tight muscles.

The pattern of radiation (or travel) of the pain can also give clues about its cause. For example, pain radiating from the back directly through to the stomach could be caused by gallbladder or pancreas problems. Pain radiating from the back down to the leg could be from numerous causes. Pain radiating to the testicles or vagina may more likely reflect a herniated disk.

Numbness is important. It can be a very frightening symptom that conjures up pictures of being crippled. Often people who have lived with back pain will first seek medical attention or start restricting their activity when their symptoms start to include numbness. Though numbness *may* indicate serious disease, often it, too, is caused by muscle tension. It is important to discuss with your doctor, but be reassured that it is most often harmless. Unfortunately, many doctors do not understand that tight muscles can cause feelings of numbness.

Your general state of health is also important, including other medical problems, medication you may be taking, and the possibility of pregnancy. You should be asked about the "red flags" (warning signs) listed in chapter 4. In addition you may be asked about the functioning of your lungs, heart, bladder, kidneys, and bowels and whether you engage in things that might expose you to serious diseases.

THE PHYSICAL EXAM

While a general physical examination is usually not critical in deducing the cause of pain, your doctor may look at structural abnormalities; the condition of the lungs, heart, or abdomen; and the circulation in the legs. If, in giving your health history, you list conditions that might signal other disease, the examination will be expanded.

Your doctor may try to see how far forward, backward, and side to side you can bend. If there has been long-standing pain, this movement is usually very restricted. A straight leg-raising test, used to test flexibility, is frequently performed. If this causes pain to radiate down the leg, it may mean a nerve is involved. If there is pain behind the knee, this usually means the muscles are tight.

One of the most important parts of the physical exam is the testing of muscle strength. Many people who have had restricted activity and pain will have mild weakness and fatigue. Marked weakness can signify nerve damage or other diseases. Symptoms like frequently dropping items even when you don't have pain, difficulty arising from a chair, tripping and falling, or catching your toes on carpet or other uneven surfaces may be more indicative of muscle weakness from neurologic causes than from deconditioning or guarding (protecting the afflicted area).

Reflexes are checked, usually at the knee and ankle. If there is a difference between left and right, it may suggest that a nerve root is being compressed. Doctors also usually scratch the bottom of the foot. An abnormal response here can mean there is a nerve problem.

Physicians check for nerve damage by noting changes in the ability to feel a pin prick or the vibration of a tuning fork. With muscle tension pain there is sometimes decreased sensation in the whole arm or leg or sometimes both the arm *and* leg on one side of the body. A skilled physician who knows about muscle or myofascial pain can usually tell whether the changes in sensation signify nerve damage.

A careful examination of the muscles may also help to identify "trigger points" or "tender points." These are places in specific muscles that are very tender when pressure is applied to them. Tenderness in certain parts of the muscles helps lead to the correct diagnosis of a muscular origin of the pain.

DIAGNOSTIC TESTS

Diagnostic tests can be very helpful to rule out serious medical disorders as the cause of chronic back pain, but they can sometimes be misleading.

BODY CHEMISTRY TESTS

Blood tests: A number of blood tests such as the *CBC* (*complete blood count*), *ESR* (*erythrocyte sedimentation rate*), and others are in common usage to screen for serious diseases that can cause or contribute to back pain.

Urinalysis: Many urinary problems can cause acute or chronic back pain. These include kidney stones, infections, blockages, or tumors. A urinalysis will come back "abnormal" in many of these conditions.

IMAGES OF THE BODY

X-rays: These are good at revealing the bony anatomy of the spine. They will show fractures, arthritis, slippage of the bones, and some tumors. X-rays do *not* show soft tissues (such as muscles, ligaments, and disks) very well; so infections, early tumors, or other medical problems will *not* be apparent on them. For the same reason, X-rays are usually not useful in diagnosing acute back pain caused by muscle problems. They can be used in cases where there has been physical trauma or if the back pain is persistent.

CAT or CT scans: *Computer-assisted tomography* is a modified X-ray. It uses X-ray radiation but augments the signal using computers and can give very clear images. It is especially useful in looking for conditions that affect the bones. It shows more about the soft tissues than simple X-rays but does not show them as well as an MRI.

MRIs: *Magnetic resonance imagery* is very commonly ordered and is excellent for showing disk, tumor, infection, or spinal cord damage. The astounding clarity and detail of MRI images can sometimes cause problems in diagnosing back pain because it becomes easy to ascribe great importance to insignificant abnormalities. There is a good chance of finding something that sounds scary on an MRI (a degenerated disk, for example) that really has nothing to do with your back problem. Many of these abnormalities are actually normal variations of anatomy, like differing eye color and nose size. Many back pain sufferers feel they cannot be properly diagnosed without an MRI. Ironically, this often results only in strengthening a false and counterproductive belief that structural damage is the cause of their pain.

Discograms: The disk has a firm outer portion called the *annulus fibrosis* and a somewhat softer inner portion called the *nucleus pulposis.* A discogram is an injection of dye into the disk, which will reveal tears in the annulus. The utility of this test is under great debate, as annular tears (like disk herniations) can be seen in people without back pain.

Bone scans: These involve an injection of radioactive dye into the blood that *may* reveal abnormalities, including infection, tumor, or arthritis. If the test is negative, many serious causes of back pain are very unlikely.

Bone density scans: This is a test used to look for osteoporosis (weakening of the bones). It is not generally used to diagnose low back pain, unless a bone has been fractured. The test can be important, since people with osteoporosis should limit the weight they lift and limit their forward bending.

Myelograms: These involve an injection of contrast material into the area around the spinal cord. This used to be the only way to see the spinal canal and nerve roots. As some risk is involved, other tests are used more commonly, particularly MRIs, though on occasion myelograms can still be of value.

IVP: *Intravenous pyelogram* is a radiologic exam of the kidneys. It is generally used to identify possible tumors or obstruction of the kidneys.

ELECTRODIAGNOSTIC TESTING (EMG)

Unlike imaging tests, which reveal structures, this test examines the *functioning* of the nerve and muscles. The EMG is quite complicated and very much dependent on the skill of the person performing it. Therefore we recommend that it be performed by a physician who is specially trained in diagnosing nerve and muscle problems and is board certified.

The test can be somewhat uncomfortable but can help distinguish the cause of pain. While imaging tests will show a disk problem in people without back pain, abnormalities on EMG are more rarely seen in people without some sort of problem or disease. In our own practice we find that this test can be quite helpful in convincing people that their pain really isn't caused by a defect in their spine.

While these and other tests help to rule out serious disorders, there is, unfortunately, no objective test to positively diagnose chronic back pain due to muscle tension. An accurate diagnosis depends on the skill and experience of the physician.

DIAGNOSIS OF CHRONIC BACK PAIN

Relevant medical diagnoses, though extremely complex, can be divided into three broad groupings, based on what is seen as the underlying cause of the problem.

SERIOUS DISEASES AND MEDICAL DISORDERS

This category involves a wide variety of possible conditions, including rheumatoid arthritis, ankylosing spondylitis (another arthritic condition), infections, tumors, ruptured aortic aneurysms (leakage in a large blood vessel), kidney stones, and osteoporosis. Though these and many other serious conditions are indeed rarely the cause of chronic back pain, they do occur, and this is the key reason that a thorough and competent medical evaluation is *absolutely essential* before beginning the Back Sense program. These are generally conditions under which undertaking an independent exercise program is not wise. Most of them call for a closely supervised medical exercise program or no exercise at all.

SERIOUS STRUCTURAL DEFECTS THAT NEED REPAIR

This category includes trauma, fracture, some severe cases of scoliosis, severe spinal stenosis, and a number of other disorders. Several of these conditions will worsen, lead to severe disability, or damage the structural integrity of the back if not treated or surgically repaired. These problems are also rare. Here again, physical exercise should be supervised by medical professionals.

Severe scoliosis: Usually *scoliosis* (excessive curvature of the spine) is minor, and people with scoliosis are no more or less likely to have back pain than the rest of the population. If the scoliosis is very pronounced (more than a thirty-degree bend), however, it can cause other problems and should be followed by a spine specialist.

Spondylolisthesis: This is a condition where one vertebra is slipping on another. Mild spondylolisthesis can be seen in people without any back pain at all. Mild to moderate spondylolisthesis does not require any special treatment or precautions. If very severe slippage is present, surgery and bracing may be needed to prevent damage to the spinal cord.

Fractures: A wide variety of bone fractures may need surgical correction or stabilization.

Spinal stenosis: *Spinal stenosis* is a condition involving narrowing of the spinal canal. This can lead to pain in the legs, particularly when walking. It sometimes needs structural repair to give the spinal cord enough room to function. It should be noted, however, that some cases of spinal stenosis respond to an exercise program with dramatic improvement. Surgery should be reserved for those individuals with progressive weakness or some cases where the pain has not responded to aggressive physical therapy. Spinal stenosis that is found with imaging tests may be unrelated to a person's back pain—some people with no pain at all show a narrowing of the spinal canal on their MRI.

MUSCULAR BACK PAIN

This category applies to the overwhelming majority of people who have chronic back pain and is the primary target of the Back Sense program. Muscular back pain is sometimes called *nonspecific back pain* or *myofascial pain*. Patients with this problem may be given diagnoses of fibromyalgia, low back strain, sacroiliac dysfunction, degenerative arthritis, bulging disks, degenerated disks, subluxations, facet joint dysfunction, and a wide variety of other labels. Often the pain associated with a diagnosis of a herniated disk is also really muscular.

People with these diagnoses may or may not demonstrate a structural abnormality. However, even if an abnormality is present, it will not worsen or pose any risk if it is not repaired. In other words, the abnormality may be simply coincidental to the back pain rather than causative. These diagnoses rarely reflect a truly serious medical condition. The pain associated with them is almost always due to the effects of muscle tension, deconditioning, and psychological conditioning. Most of the time there is no need to adjust your activity because you were given one of these diagnoses, and exercise is an appropriate part of treatment.

Myofascial pain: This diagnosis implies that certain muscles are causing the pain. This can be determined by *palpation* (exerting pressure on the muscle) in specific areas. Finding the exact muscle or sets of muscles that are particularly tender can help to tailor an activity program to get the most pain relief. Many times the exact pain symptoms and symptoms of numbness or tingling can be reproduced by firm pressure on the muscle. It can be very reassuring to the patient to know where the pain is coming from and to realize there is no nerve damage.

Disk problems: These represent an entire class of very common diagnoses made by medical doctors and chiropractors. In a great number of cases, back pain is completely unrelated to the damaged disk. Because these diagnoses are so prevalent, and so many people are concerned about them, we want to describe them in some detail:

Degenerative disk disease refers to normal changes in disks. As they age, disks lose some moisture and elasticity. The spaces between the bones in the spine may become smaller. The disks themselves cannot be seen on an X-ray, but their condition can be inferred from the distance between the bones in the spine. An MRI easily reveals the amount of water in the disk. Degenerative disk disease is very common but generally *does not* produce back pain. Therefore, even if degenerated disks are found, it is quite unlikely that they are the *cause* of pain. The diagnosis tends to strike people as being ominous, however, and often conjures up images of gradual deterioration and disability. Disk degeneration is best considered an inconsequential part of the normal aging process.

Bulging disk is another diagnosis that often causes worry but is usually insignificant. It means that a disk is bulging beyond the bony vertebra.

Over 60 percent of people *without any* back pain will have some disk abnormality such as a bulge.

Diskogenic pain and *annular tears* are terms used to describe a disk that has a tear in the firm outer surface, but no disk material has protruded out from the disk. Though we know that disks are capable of generating pain, the frequency of annular tears has been shown to be equal in patients with and without back pain.

Disk herniation and *radiculopathy* are diagnoses that *may* identify a real, yet rare, cause of back pain. Theses diagnoses are used much too frequently, however, and are often based primarily on an MRI or CAT finding or on pain that travels down the leg. Discovering a disk herniation on MRI is very common in people *without* any back or leg pain whatsoever. Symptoms, or test findings, that *are* consistent with a disk herniation include significantly worse pain in the legs than in the back; loss of sensation in a certain area; loss of proper reflexes; loss of strength; increase in pain upon coughing, sneezing, or bowel movements; and pain radiating down the leg that burns or hurts during a special flexibility test. If several of these signs are not present, you may still have a disk herniation, but it is unlikely that the disk herniation is causing your back pain.

Unfortunately, many physicians assume that sciatica (pain down the leg) is always caused by a disk problem. It is very important to realize that most sciatica, like most back pain, is actually caused by tightness of muscles. The nerves that produce sensations in the legs pass through and near many muscles in the buttocks and the legs themselves. Tension and reduced blood flow in these muscles readily lead to sensations of pain, tingling, or numbness in the legs or feet. Finding the trigger point that can reproduce this pain down the leg can be very reassuring and help to start the process of recovery. In most patients with an initial diagnosis of disk-related pain, we can find a muscular source for the pain.

Fibromyalgia: This condition involves long-standing pain problems, generalized pain in more than one area of the body, and an increased sensitivity to pressure over certain pressure points. The sufferer will often describe feeling bad in general, difficulty with sleep, and being poorly rested. People with fibromyalgia will often have low back pain or neck pain as a very prominent feature of their symptoms, although they will also have pain in many other areas. Since the pain is muscular, it can be treated using the Back Sense program.

Low back strain: This is a broad diagnosis and usually indicates that there is nothing structurally wrong with the back. The term itself is a little misleading, as one would usually expect a strain to get better over a short period of time and this term is used for chronic back pain.

Arthritis: This is a diagnosis similar to disk degeneration. Arthritis means inflammation of a joint, usually with pain and changes in its structure. Structural changes of the spine are very commonly found on X-rays, especially as one ages. However, there are many cases where people have no back pain, yet arthritis is found on an X-ray. There are situations when the arthritis *is* causing the back pain, but this is much rarer than many practitioners think. In these unusual cases, medications *are* usually effective, certain activities are reliably associated with the pain, and rest generally relieves it. In treating muscular pain, medicines are generally not helpful, activities are only variably associated with pain, and rest is not helpful.

Rheumatoid arthritis generally necessitates a little more caution in exercise than osteoarthritis. Rheumatoid arthritis can cause significant changes in the joints and is more likely to lead to instability than osteoarthritis. Your doctor should easily be able to distinguish the type of arthritis that you have.

Sacroiliac dysfunction: This is a diagnosis used by physical therapists, chiropractors and osteopathic physicians. There is widespread belief among them that misalignment of the pelvis can lead to back pain, and entire treatment regimens are based upon this idea. A number of the treatments for it have proven to be no more effective than a placebo in relieving pain. The misalignment is usually due to muscle tension.

Subluxation: This is a term commonly used by chiropractors for what they feel is at the root of much back pain. They believe that slight misalignments of the spine cause many problems, involving pain or other body dysfunction. Many of their treatments are meant to adjust these misalignments. These theories are highly controversial and, like many other theories about the cause of back pain, have little research support to back them up.

TMS: *Tension myositis syndrome* is a diagnosis used by Dr. John Sarno and some other practitioners. This diagnosis is similar to myofascial pain.

APPENDIX 2

MEDICAL TREATMENT OF BACK PAIN

A remarkable number of treatments are available for back pain. Unfortunately this can lead to overwhelming options, with no clear indication as to which is best. Many people describe frustration with differing opinions as to what will most effectively alleviate the discomfort. The huge variety of possible treatments can also make it difficult to determine when to discontinue one and try another.

The best explanation for such a large range of treatments is that most (including no treatment at all) work a good deal of the time, yet none work in every case. A review by a leading researcher in the *New England Journal of Medicine* concluded that doctors and patients "fall prey to successive fads" of back pain treatment that result in considerable unnecessary pain and expense. Many treatments may be harmful in that they tend to reinforce the erroneous idea that there is a physical remedy for the pain, rather than emphasizing the change in understanding and behavior that is needed to make true progress.

MEDICATIONS

Numerous medicines are used in the treatment of acute and chronic pain. Many of them are employed despite a lack of scientific evidence for their effectiveness. While medications can be helpful at times, they are probably overused by most doctors.

It is therefore important to clearly think through decisions to use medicines. Many can cloud thinking, disturb sleep, aggravate depression, and create physical dependence. In chapter 11 we offer suggestions for dealing with these potential drawbacks of medications.

Nonsteroidal anti-inflammatory medications (NSAIDs): These are very commonly used in treating back pain. They reduce inflammation and lessen pain. They are generally fairly safe in the short run but do have some potentially serious long-term side effects. They may help in reducing the pain from a new injury but are typically not effective for older injuries (those that occurred more than two weeks ago) or for alleviating chronic pain. Some of these medications are now available without a prescription. Common examples include aspirin, ibuprofen (Motrin, Advil), naproxen (Aleve, Anaprox), Orudis, Daypro, Toradol, Vioxx, and Celebrex.

Acetaminophen (Tylenol): This nonprescription pain reliever is safe for most people when used as directed. It doesn't reduce inflammation but is as effective as the NSAIDs in reducing pain from other sources and generally has fewer side effects. It is fine to use during acute pain, but long-term use can cause liver or kidney problems. It is also sold under many other brands and as a "non-aspirin pain reliever."

Muscle relaxants: These are widely used for acute injuries. They are generally safe, though they often cause significant fatigue and are only intermittently effective. Some are related to the antidepressant medications. Common medications in this group include cyclobenzaprine (Flexeril) and Robaxin. The antianxiety medicines described below are also often prescribed as muscle relaxants.

Narcotics: These are less widely employed, and there is quite a bit of variation in how they are used to treat back pain. They do not affect the nerve signals from the muscles but change how the pain is perceived in the brain. They are without question the most effective medications available for acute pain but have the serious disadvantage of being physically and psychologically habit-forming. Taken over time, they produce both *tolerance,* in which more and more of the drug is needed to have the same effect; and *dependency,* in which withdrawal symptoms occur if the drug is suddenly discontinued. The fact that drug addicts often use complaints of back pain to obtain narcotics has led many doctors to refuse to prescribe them for the problem. Typical drugs in this category include Darvon or Darvocet, Vicodin, Percodan, Percocet, and Demerol. In our view these drugs rarely have *any* place in the treatment of chronic low back pain, since they interfere with restoring normal activity.

Antidepressant medications: These medications have been in widespread use for many years to treat a number of psychological and physical problems, including serious depression and some cases of neurologically caused pain. They do not appear to be useful for acute pain treatment, but some of the older *tricyclic antidepressants,* such as amitriptyline (Elavil) and nortriptyline, may help reduce long-term pain when used in low doses. Their effectiveness as a treatment for chronic pain is quite variable and seems to diminish with time for some people. While all antidepressant medicines have side effects, a group called *SSRIs* (*selective serotonin reuptake inhibitors*) have significantly fewer side effects than earlier antidepressants and are now most commonly used to help with depression. The most widely known of these include Prozac, Zoloft, Paxil, Celexa, and Luvox. Other types of antidepressants that are more appropriate for some people include Effexor, Wellbutrin, Serzone, trazodone, and Remeron. Some antidepressants are helpful for insomnia.

Antianxiety medications: The intense and persistent anxiety that may be associated with chronic back pain can be helped, in some cases, by psychiatric medicines. A group of medicines called *benzodiazepines,* of which Valium, Librium, Xanax, Klonopin, Serax, and Ativan are well-known examples, reduce anxiety, muscle tension, and the fight-or-flight response very effectively for short periods of time. Unfortunately they can also make us less alert, interfere with concentration, and readily become habit-forming. Many who take these drugs for more than a short period become physically and psychologically dependent upon them. This can be problematic, for a common symptom of benzodiazepine withdrawal is an increase in feelings of anxiety, which will, of course, tempt people to take more of the drug. Generally these medicines are best used for brief periods of extreme stress or for short-term treatment of insomnia. Having them available for emergencies can also offer the reassurance that if our anxiety ever felt completely overwhelming, we'd have a way to deal with it.

The SSRIs mentioned above are not habit-forming and can also reduce anxiety, including the intense waves of anxiety that manifest as panic attacks. There are also other medicines, such as *buspirone* (BuSpar), that are not habit-forming and reduce generalized anxiety.

While medications have their place in helping people with serious anxiety, and are useful during crises, we advise against using them routinely as a long-term strategy for working with the anxiety connected to chronic back pain. Most people struggling with this can benefit far more from techniques aimed at identifying underlying emotions that are contributing to anxiety and gradually facing feared situations. Aerobic exercise, stretching, and mindfulness routines can also make anxiety manageable for many people.

INJECTIONS

Epidural steroid injections: These are commonly used if there is evidence of a radiculopathy. They involve injecting steroid medications into the back near where the nerve is presumably being pressed and may be used one to three times. If the pain is actually caused by a disk herniation, the injections can temporarily decrease discomfort, though an aggressive return to activity is still needed. We will sometimes use these injections for temporary relief if we are convinced a disk herniation is causing the pain. Studies of the general effectiveness of epidural steroid injections as a treatment for back pain have not been encouraging.

Trigger point injections: These usually consist of short-acting anesthetic medication injected into a muscle at the point where it hurts. They may very temporarily ease the discomfort in the muscle and allow a person to stretch farther; but trigger point injections by themselves do not appear to be an effective treatment. As an alternative for mild, temporary pain relief, we usually encourage the use of hot or cold packs and stretches. The injections may be helpful if they are followed immediately by stretching and if they are gradually decreased, but we do not use them in our own practice.

Facet injections: These are injections of either steroids or anesthetics into the facet joints (the connections between adjoining vertebrae). They are based on the diagnosis of arthritis in these joints. This diagnosis is frequently questionable, as the condition is often merely coincidental to the pain. Up to three injections may be used, but this should be coupled with a physical rehabilitation program. In our own practice we use these injections very rarely, as research on their effectiveness has been discouraging.

SURGERY

There is a wide variety of surgeries available for back pain. While these may very rarely be necessary, a proper diagnosis is very important since there is an unfortunately common problem called the *failed back surgery syndrome*. It describes people who have had one or more surgeries but persist in having severe pain. Many surgeons will give only fifty-fifty odds of success for back surgery. The poor and unpredictable results of surgery have frustrated all concerned and reflect the fact that surgery is performed routinely on many patients who are not likely to benefit from it.

Disk surgery: In the unlikely case that a disk herniation really is the cause of the pain, surgery may make you feel better sooner, though you may wish to simply wait it out, since the pain from herniations will also usually get better without surgery. This can be true even for very large herniations. The typical surgery for a disk herniation is called a *diskectomy.* It is important to realize that except for rare, serious problems, such as *cauda equina syndrome,* which causes bladder and bowel dysfunction, such disk surgery need not be done immediately. There is almost always plenty of time to try other methods first.

Spinal fusions: This is a major operation that takes bone from the pelvis and inserts it into the spine to create a more rigid structure. It is sometimes offered to patients with back pain. Unfortunately the proof that this works better than a placebo is scarce. The complications for this surgery, though infrequent, can be horrendous, and the expense is huge. Though we will send a rare patient for a diskectomy, we almost never refer patients for spinal fusion.

OTHER TREATMENTS

Braces and corsets: These are prescribed to reduce strain on back muscles or to protect supposedly weak or damaged structures. They are almost always harmful, since they limit normal movement, worsen muscle deconditioning, and reinforce the idea that your back is damaged and needs protection.

TENS and PENS: *TENS* (*transcutaneous electrical nerve stimulation*) and more recently *PENS* (*percutaneous electrical nerve stimulation*) treatments are often used for chronic pain. TENS involves delivering tiny electric shocks from the surface of the skin, while PENS uses small needles to deliver the shocks. Both seem to work by drawing our attention away from pain sensations. While they can temporarily distract us from intense pain, they do little to relieve the muscle tension that creates most chronic back pain.

Hot and cold packs: These are often suggested as a way of managing acute pain, and many people report relief from using them. They can be effective for brief periods of time to relieve intense discomfort.

Commercial hot water bottles, heating pads, and ice packs are readily available in drugstores. A bag of frozen peas also works well as a cold pack. We recommend them for people who are troubled by increases in pain that may initially accompany stretching and exercise. It is important, however, not to become preoccupied with relieving pain.

Physical therapy: Many varieties of physical therapy are used to treat both acute and chronic pain. Based on clinical experience, we feel that very aggressive and active therapy can hasten recovery from *acute* back pain, though this has not yet been proven by research. Aggressive therapy is especially valuable in treating *chronic* back pain, particularly if there is a loss of range of motion or strength, and this *has* been well demonstrated in scientific studies. Any good physical therapy program should include stretching, strengthening, and aerobic conditioning. The *passive* electrical stimulation, heat, ultrasound, or traction methods that are sometimes employed by physical therapists may have a place in treatment of acute back pain (to temporarily reduce the pain if coupled with exercise), but they do not appear to have any value in treating chronic pain.

Chiropractic treatment: Chiropractors treat a wide variety of back disorders. They use spinal manipulation and theorize that misalignment of the spine causes many pain problems. They also believe that misaligned vertebrae can be manually put back into place. Chiropractic treatment may help for acute episodes of back pain but is generally not effective for chronic pain. While the treatment may relax some muscles and help you to feel that something is being done, most chiropractors reinforce the counterproductive idea that there is a problem with the structure of the back. In addition many chiropractors will discourage activities that cause pain.

Massage: Massage is similar to chiropractic treatment in that it may provide some immediate pain relief. Often the pain will recur if the massage is not coupled with aggressive stretching. Massage does have the benefit of helping you to feel what it is like to have your muscles relax, at least temporarily. There are a number of different massage styles, but there is no scientific indication that one is better than another.

Acupuncture: This is an ancient Asian form of treatment that involves the use of fine needles placed in specific locations. Some people find it effective temporarily in reducing pain and anxiety.

Please tell us about your experiences with *Back Sense* and chronic back pain. The information will be used to help others and to refine the program. To contact us, visit our website: backsense.org.

APPENDIX 3

RESOURCES

PART I: UNDERSTANDING CHRONIC BACK PAIN

Medical resources for more information on back pain:

The *Agency for Health Care Policy and Research Guideline* is a very authoritative treatise on diagnosis and treatment of acute back pain with an extensive list of original scientific articles. It is available in three forms: the full clinical practice guideline, which includes all the references; the quick reference guide for clinicians (for health care professionals, though this is also a good review for the interested and knowledgeable layperson); and the consumers' guide.

It is available on the Web by going to http://text.nlm.nih.gov/ftrs/dbaccess/ahcpr.

Once you have reached this site you need to fill in the blanks and select *14. Acute Low Back Problems in Adults.* Navigation is a little tricky but worthwhile. By mail the guideline can be ordered from the Government Printing Office, Superintendent of Documents, Washington, DC 20402; (202) 512–1800.

Bigos, S.; Bowyer, O.; Braen, G.; et al. Acute Low Back Problems in Adults. Clinical Practice Guideline No. 14. AHCPR Publication No. 95–0642. Rockville, MD: Agency for Health Care Policy and Research, Public Health Service, U.S. Department of Health and Human Services. December 1994.

An excellent review of medical diagnosis and treatment of back pain. Also has a very good section on finding a doctor and questions to ask a doctor:

Sinel, M. S.; Deardorff, W. W.; Goldstein, T. B. Win the battle against back pain: An integrated mind-body approach. New York: Dell; 1996.

Additional help in finding a doctor:

The American Academy of Physical Medicine and Rehabilitation can help you find a physiatrist in your area. This can be done through their Web site (www.aapmr.org) or by contacting them at American Academy of Physical Medicine and Rehabilitation, One IBM Plaza, Suite 2500, Chicago, IL 60611–3604; phone (312) 464–9700; fax (312) 464–0227.

Detailed description of the structure of the back:

Sinel, M. S.; Deardorff, W. W.; Goldstein, T. B. Win the battle against back pain: An integrated mind-body approach. New York: Dell; 1996.

Excellent, readable review of scientific literature about the stress response:

Sapolsky, R. M. Why zebras don't get ulcers: An updated guide to stress, stress-related diseases, and coping. New York: W. H. Freeman Co.; 1998.

Other books on the effects of stress with an emphasis on stress management:

Benson, H.; Klipper, M. Z. The relaxation response. New York: Avon Books; 2000.

Benson, H.; Stark, M. Timeless healing: The power and biology of belief. New York: Simon & Schuster; 1996.

Borysenko, J. Minding the body, mending the mind. New York: Dell; 1993.

Domar, A. D.; Dreher, H. Healing mind, healthy woman: Using the mind-body connection to manage stress and take control of your life. New York: H. Holt & Co.; 1996.

Goleman, D.; Gurin, J. (ed). Mind and body medicine: How to use your mind for better health, vol. 1. Yonkers, NY: Consumer Reports Books; 1993.

Ornstein, R.; Swenciionis, C. (eds.). The healing brain: A scientific reader. New York: Guilford Press; 1990:69.

A comprehensive review of the placebo effect:

Harrington, A. (ed). The placebo effect: An interdisciplinary exploration. Boston, MA: Harvard University Press; 1997.

A somewhat different approach to back pain treatment, which also views it as a tension-related disorder. Dr. Sarno is one of the primary originators of this treatment approach:

Sarno, J. Healing back pain: The mind-body connection. New York: Warner Books; 1991.

Sarno, J. The Mindbody prescription: Healing the body, healing the pain. New York: Warner Books; 1998.

PART II: RELIEVING CHRONIC BACK PAIN

Working with angry feelings in relationships:

Lerner, H. G. The dance of anger: A woman's guide to changing the patterns of intimate relationships. New York: Harper & Row; 1985.

Learning to be more assertive:

Bower, S. A.; Bower, G. H. Asserting yourself: A practical guide for positive change. Reading, MA: Addison-Wesley; 1976.

Using journal writing to work with emotions:

Pennebaker, J. W. Opening up: The healing power of expressing emotions. New York: Guilford Press; 1997.

For help with sexual problems:

Barbach, L. B. For yourself: The fulfillment of female sexuality. New York: Anchor/Doubleday; 1976.

Zilbergeld, B. The new male sexuality: The truth about men, sex, and pleasure. New York: Bantam; 1999.

Good general introductions to meditation practice:

Roche, L. Meditation made easy. New York: HarperCollins; 1998.

Bodian, S. Meditation for dummies. Foster City, CA: IDG Books; 1999.

Good guide to practicing mindfulness in daily life:

Kabat-Zinn, J. Wherever you go, there you are: Mindfulness meditation in everyday life. New York: Hyperion; 1995.

An excellent resource on stress, exercise, diet, insomnia, and general wellness and disease prevention:

Benson, H.; Stuart, E. M. The wellness book: The comprehensive guide to maintaining health and treating stress-related illness. New York: Simon & Schuster; 1992.

Additional resource on exercise:

American College of Sports Medicine (ACSM) Fitness Book, 2nd edition, American College of Sports Medicine. Champaign, IL: Human Kinetics; 1998 (Web site: www.acsm.org).

Additional resource site:

www.WebMD.com

Videos are also a good way to learn more about fitness and exercise. For increasing flexibility and learning more about mindful stretching, yoga tapes are useful. For endurance training, you can find aerobics tapes at varying levels of intensity.

Personal trainers and gyms are also good sources for information on exercise.

REFERENCES

CHAPTER 1

Research demonstrating very low incidence of serious medical disease as a cause of back pain:

Bigos, S.; Bowyer, O.; Braen, G.; et al. Acute low back problems in adults. Clinical Practice Guideline No. 14. AHCPR Publication No. 95–0642. Rockville, MD: Agency for Health Care Policy and Research, Public Health Service, U.S. Department of Health and Human Services. December 1994.

Deyo, R. A.; Diehl, A. K.; Cancer as a cause of back pain: Frequency, clinical presentation, and diagnostic strategies. *Journal of General Internal Medicine* 3 (3; May–June 1988): 230–38.

Deyo, R. A.; Rainville, J.; Kent, D. L. What can the history and physical examination tell us about low back pain? *JAMA* 268 (6; Aug. 12, 1992): 760–65.

Waddell, G.; Main, C. J.; Morris, E. W.; Venner, R. M.; Rae, P. S.; Sharmy, S. H.; Galloway, H. Normality and reliability in the clinical assessment of backache. *British Medical Journal* (Clinical Research Edition) 284 (6328; May 22, 1982): 1519–23.

Dr. John Sarno's treatment methods (discussed in story):

Sarno, J. *Healing back pain: The mind-body connection.* New York: Warner Books, 1991.

Sarno, J. *The Mindbody prescription: Healing the body, healing the pain.* New York: Warner Books, 1998.

CHAPTER 3

Back pain usually appears "out of the blue":

Hall, H.; McIntosh, G.; Wilson, L.; Melles, T. Spontaneous onset of back pain. *Clinical Journal of Pain* 14 (2; June 1998): 129–33.

Structural "abnormalities" are found in people without pain. Study described in the *New England Journal of Medicine:*

Jensen, M. C.; Brant-Zawadzki, M. D.; Obucowski, N.; Modic, M. T.; Malkasian, D.; Ross, J. S. Magnetic resonance imaging of the lumbar spine in people without back pain. *New England Journal of Medicine* 331 (2; July 14, 1994): 69–73.

A few of the many other studies showing widespread structural "abnormalities" in pain-free subjects:

Boden, S. D.; Davis, D. O.; Dina, T. S.; Patronas, N. J.; Wiesel, S. W. Abnormal magnetic-resonance scans of the lumbar spine in asymptomatic subjects. A prospective investigation. *Journal of Bone and Joint Surgery* (American Edition) 72 (3; Mar. 1990): 403–8.

Stadnik, T. W.; Lee, R. R.; Coen, H. L.; Neirynck, E. C.; Buisseret, T. S.;

Osteaux, M. J. Annular tears and disk herniation: prevalence and contrast enhancement on MR images in the absence of low back pain or sciatica. *Radiology* 206 (1998): 4–55.

Wiesel, S. W.; Tsourmas, N.; Feffer, H. L.; Citrin, C. M.; Patronas, N. A study of computer-assisted tomography. I. The incidence of positive CAT scans in an asymptomatic group of patients. *Spine* 9 (6; Sept. 1984): 549–51.

Patients with back pain who have no clear structural abnormality when tested:

Frymoyer, J. W. Back pain and sciatica. *New England Journal of Medicine* 318 (5; Feb. 4, 1988): 291–300.

MRI study of patients one year after surgery showing no consistent relationship between the state of their disk and current pain level:

Tullberg, T.; Grane, P.; Isacson, J. Gadolinium-enhanced magnetic resonance imaging of 36 patients one year after lumbar disc resection. *Spine* 19 (2; Jan. 15, 1994): 176–82.

MRI study ten years after surgery where over a third still had herniated disks, but this had no bearing on whether or not they had pain:

Fraser, R. D.; Sandhu, A.; Gogan, W. J. Magnetic resonance imaging findings ten years after treatment for lumbar disc herniation. *Spine* 20 (6; Mar. 15, 1995): 710–14.

Review of medical records of surgeries that found nothing out of place but were followed by relief almost half the time:

Spangforte, E. V. The lumbar disk herniation: A computer-aided analysis of 2504 operations. *Acta Orthopaedica Scandinavica* 142 (Supp.; 1972): 1–95.

Review of medical literature showing that poor, rural farmers have much less back pain than people in developed countries:

Volinn, E. The epidemiology of low back pain in the rest of the world. A review of surveys in low-middle-income countries. *Spine* 22 (15; Aug. 1, 1997): 1747–54.

Back pain disability is rare in developing countries, probably owing to different cultural attitudes:

Sinel, M. S.; Deardorff, W. W.; Goldstein, T. B. *Win the battle against back pain: An integrated mind-body approach.* New York: Dell, 1996, pp. 45–46.

Study showing widely disparate rates of back surgery and other procedures in different U.S. cities (sidebar):

In the U.S., all medicine is local. *New York Times*, Feb. 4, 1996.

It takes time for doctors to adopt up-to-date treatments:

The long shelf life of medical myths. *New York Times*, Dec. 5, 1996.

Outdated views on ulcers hinder cures. *New York Times*, May 25, 1999.

CHAPTER 4

Very low incidence of serious medical causes of back pain, red flags for diagnosing serious diseases:

Bigos, S.; Bowyer, O.; Braen, G.; et al. Acute low back problems in adults. Clinical Practice Guideline No. 14. AHCPR Publication No. 95–0642. Rockville, MD: Agency for Health Care Policy and Research, Public Health Service, U.S. Department of Health and Human Services. December 1994.

It is safe to exercise if you do not have a serious medical cause of pain:

Mayer, T. G.; Gatchel, R. J.; Mayer, H.; Kishino, N. D.; Keeley, J.; Mooney, V. A prospective two-year study of functional restoration in industrial low back injury: An objective assessment procedure [published erratum appears in *JAMA* 259 (2; Jan. 8, 1988): 220]. *JAMA* 258 (13; Oct. 2, 1987); 1763–66.

CHAPTER 5

Boeing study showing that psychological stress was more important than physical factors in predicting who developed back pain:

Bigos, S. J.; Battie, M. C.; Spengler, D. M.; Fisher, L. D.; Fordyce, W. E.; Hansson, T. H.; Nachemson, A. L.; Wortley, M. D. A prospective study of work perceptions and psychosocial factors affecting the report of back injury [published erratum appears in *Spine* 16 (6; June 1991): 688]. *Spine* 16 (1; Jan. 1991): 1–6.

Examples of the many other studies from around the world linking back pain to psychological stress at work:

Ahlberg-Hulten, G. K.; Theorell, T.; Sigala, F. Social support, job strain and musculoskeletal pain among female health care personnel. *Scandinavian Journal of Work, Environment and Health* 21 (6; Dec. 1995): 435–39 (Sweden).

Papageorgiou, A. C.; Macfarlane, G. J.; Thomas, E.; Croft, P. R.; Jayson, M. I.; Silman, A. J. Psychosocial factors in the workplace—do they predict new episodes of low back pain? Evidence from the South Manchester Back Pain Study. *Spine* 22 (10; May 15, 1997): 1137–42 (Britain).

Van Poppel, M. N. M.; Koes, B. W.; Deville, W.; Smid, T.; Bouter, L. M.; Risk factors for back pain incidence in industry: A prospective study. *Pain* 77 (1; July 1998): 81–86 (Netherlands).

Williams, R. A.; Pruitt, S. D.; Doctor, J. N.; Epping-Jordan, J. E.; Wahlgren, D. R.; Grand, I.; Patterson, T. L.; Webster, J. S.; Slater, J. A.; Atkinson, J. H. The contribution of job satisfaction to the transition from acute to chronic low-back pain. *Archives of Physical Medicine and Rehabilitation* 79 (1998): 366–75 (U.S.A.).

Examples of studies showing that other psychological stressors lead to back pain:

Raising kids is a pain in the . . . *The Back Letter* 9 (12; Dec. 1994): 140.

Back pain under fire: Do police in a war zone suffer an increased risk of back problems? *The Back Letter* 11 (10; Oct. 1996): 111.

Lampe, A.; Stollner, W.; Krismer, M.; Rumpold, G.; Kantner-Rumplmair, W.; Ogon, M.; Rathner, G. The impact of stressful life events on exacerbation of chronic low-back pain. *Journal of Psychosomatic Research* 44 (5; May 1998): 555–63.

Examples of reviews of medical literature indicating the many health problems caused by stress:

For professionals:

Gatchel, R. J.; Blanchard, E. B. (eds.). *Psychophysiological disorders: Research and clinical applications.* Washington, DC.: American Psychological Association, 1993.

For laypeople:

Domar, A. D.; Dreher, H. *Healing mind, healthy woman: Using the mind-body connection to manage stress and take control of your life.* New York: Henry Holt & Co., 1996.

Goleman, D.; Gurin, J. (eds). *Mind and body medicine: How to use your mind for better health, vol. 1.* Yonkers, NY: Consumer Reports Books, 1993.

Sapolsky, R. M. *Why zebras don't get ulcers: An updated guide to stress, stress-related diseases, and coping.* New York: W. H. Freeman Co., 1998.

Stress makes wounds heal more slowly:

Kiecolt-Glaser, J. K.; Page, G. G.; Marucha, P. T.; MacCallum, R. C.; Glaser, R. Psychological influences on surgical recovery: Perspectives from psychoneuroimmunology. *American Psychologist* 53 (11; Nov. 1998): 1209–18.

Case of woman whose nausea was cured by syrup of ipecac (normally used to induce vomiting):

Wolf, S. Effect of suggestion and psychological conditioning on the act of chemical agents in human subjects: The pharmacology of placebos. *Journal of Clinical Investigation* 29 (1950): 10–109.

Blood pressure responded powerfully to expectations:

Agras, W. S.; Horne, M.; Taylor, C. B. Expectation and the blood-pressure-lowering effects of relaxation. *Psychosomatic Medicine* 44 (4; Sept. 1982): 389–95.

Studies showing that seemingly effective surgical "cure" for angina pectoris was actually a placebo response:

Cobb, L. A.; Thomas, G. I.; Dillard, D. H.; Merendino, K. A.; Bruce, R. A. An evaluation of internal-mammary-artery-ligation by a double-blind technic. *New England Journal of Medicine* 260 (1959): 1115–18.

Dimond, E. G.; Kittle, C. F.; Crockett, J. E. Comparison of internal mammary ligation and sham operation for angina pectoris. *American Journal of Cardiology* (5; 1960): 483–86.

Sham tooth grinding cured TMJ symptoms 64 percent of the time:

Goodman, P.; Greene, C. S.; Laskin, D. M. Response of patients with myofascial pain-dysfunction syndrome to mock equilibration. *Journal of the American Dental Association* 92 (1976): 755–58.

Placebos have extensive negative side effects:

Turner, J. A.; Deyo, R. A.; Loeser, J. D.; Von Korff, M.; Fordyce, W. E. The importance of placebo effects in pain treatment and research. *JAMA* 271 (20; May 25, 1994): 1609–13.

CHAPTER 6

Vast majority of acute back pain episodes heal themselves within a month or two without special treatment:

Waddell, G. 1987 Volvo award in clinical sciences: A new clinical model for the treatment of low-back pain. *Spine* 12 (7; Sept. 1987): 632–44.

Back pain often starts "out of the blue":

See citation in chapter 3, Hall.

Study showing that many anxiety- and tension-related problems that appear to come from "out of the blue" actually follow emotionally upsetting events that we don't connect to them:

Vuksic-Mihaljevic, Z.; Mandic, N.; Barkic, J.; Mrdenovic, S. A current psychodynamic understanding of panic disorder. *British Journal of Medical Psychology* 71 (Pt. 1; Mar. 1998): 27–45.

Study with four different exercises showing that back pain patients in particular show increased back muscle tension when talking about emotionally upsetting events:

Flor, H.; Turk, D. C.; Birbaumer, N. Assessment of stress-related psychophysiological reactions in chronic back pain patients. *Journal of Consulting and Clinical Psychology* 53 (3; June 1985): 354–64.

Additional studies demonstrating that people with back pain tense their back muscles when emotionally stressed more than others do:

DeGood, D. E.; Stewart, W. R.; Adams, L. E.; Dale, J. A. Paraspinal EMG and autonomic reactivity of patients with back pain and controls to personally relevant stress. *Perceptual and Motor Skills* 79 (3, Pt. 1; Dec. 1994): 1399–1409.

Dickson-Parnell, B.; Zeichner, A. The premenstrual syndrome: psychophysiologic concomitants of perceived stress and low back pain. *Pain* 34 (2; Aug. 1998): 161–69.

People specifically tense the area where they generally suffer pain, but not other areas, when emotionally stressed:

Flor, H.; Birbaumer, N.; Schugens, M. M.; Lutzenberger, W. Symptom-specific psychophysiological responses in chronic pain patients. *Psychophysiology* 29 (4; July 1992): 452–60.

Depression is three to four times more frequent in people with chronic back pain than in the general population:

Sullivan, M. J.; Reesor, K.; Mikail, S.; Fisher, R. The treatment of depression in chronic low back pain: Review and recommendations. *Pain* 50 (1; July 1992): 5–13.

As many as 92 percent of people with chronic back pain have at least mild depression:

Swami, D. R.; Nathawat, S. S.; Vyas, J. M.; Upadhyay, J. P. Depression and chronic low back pain. *Indian Journal of Clinical Psychology* 18 (1; Mar. 1991): 35–36.

Freud's famous 1917 paper describing how anger turned against the self causes depression:

Freud, S. Mourning and Melancholia. In Strachey, J. (ed). *The standard edition of the complete psychological works of Sigmund Freud.* Vol. XIV. London: The Hogart Press, 1974.

Examples of recent scientific studies showing a connection between holding anger in and depression:

Begley, T. M. Expressed and suppressed anger as predictors of health complaints. *Journal of Organizational Behavior* 15 (6; Nov. 1994): 503–16.

Brody, C. L.; Haaga, D. A. F.; Kirk, L.; Solomon, A. Experiences of anger in people who have recovered from depression and never-depressed people. *Journal of Nervous and Mental Disease* 187 (7; July 1999): 400–5.

Tschannen, T. A.; Duckro, P. N.; Margolis, R. B.; Tomazic, T. J. The relationship of anger, depression, and perceived disability among headache patients. *Headache* 32 (10; Nov. 1992): 501–3.

Research on developing learned helplessness (sidebar):

Seligman, M. E. P. *Helplessness: On depression, development, and death. A series of books in psychology.* San Francisco: W. H. Freeman, 1975.

CHAPTER 7

Examples of research showing that fear of activity and fear of pain, rather than pain itself, leads to disability:

Crombez, G.; Vlaeyen, J. W. S.; Heuts, P. H. T. G.; Lysens, R. Pain-related fear is more disabling than pain itself: Evidence on the role of pain-related fear in chronic back pain disability. *Pain* 80 (1–2; Mar. 1999): 329–39.

Waddell, G.; Newton, M.; Henderson, I.; Somerville, D. A fear-avoidance beliefs questionnaire (FABQ) and the role of fear-avoidance beliefs in chronic low back pain and disability. *Pain* 52 (2; Feb. 1993): 157–68.

Programs of vigorous activity reduce pain by 50 percent without even addressing the role of stress:

Rainville, J.; Sobel, J. B.; Hartigan, C.; Wright, A. The effect of compensation involvement on the reporting of pain and disability by patients referred for rehabilitation of chronic low back pain. *Spine* 22 (17; Sept. 1, 1997): 2016–24.

Workers with acute back pain who were encouraged not to rest but to continue normal activity had the best outcomes:

Malmivaara, A.; Hakkinen, U.; Aro, T.; Heinrichs, M. L.; Koskenniemi, L.; Kuosma, E.; Lappi, S.; Paloheimo, R.; Servo, C.; Vaaranen, V.; et al. The treatment of acute low back pain—bed rest, exercises, or ordinary activity? [See comments.] *New England Journal of Medicine* 332 (6; Feb. 9, 1995): 351–55.

Subjects assigned to two days of bed rest returned to work 45 percent sooner than those who rested for seven days:

Deyo, R. A.; Diehl, A. K.; Rosenthat, M. How many days of bed rest for acute low back pain? A randomized clinical trial. *New England Journal of Medicine* 315 (17; Oct. 23, 1986): 1064–70.

Systematic review of studies showing that normal activity is superior to rest for acute back pain:

Waddell, G.; Feder, G.; Lewis, M. Systematic reviews of bed rest and advice to stay active for acute low back pain. *British Journal of General Practice* 47 (423; Oct. 1997): 647–52.

Large study showing that vigorous exercise was far superior to conventional treatments for helping people to recover from back pain and return to work.

Mitchell, R. I.; Carmen, G. M. Results of a multicenter trial using an intensive active exercise program for the treatment of acute soft tissue and back injuries. *Spine* 15 (6; June 1990): 514–21.

Study showing that patients could significantly improve their physical capacity without any significant increase in pain, even though they believed that the exercises would cause more pain:

Rainville, J.; Ahern, D. K.; Phalen, L.; Childs, L. A.; Sutherland, R. The association of pain with physical activities in chronic low back pain. *Spine* 17 (9; Sept. 1992): 1060–64.

Study of four thousand postal workers that showed no benefit from extensive back school program that included professional training in back safety:

Daltroy, L. H.; Iversen, M. D., Larson, M. G.; Lew, R.; Wright, E.; Ryan, J.; Zwerling, C.; Fossel, A. H.; Liang, M. H. A controlled trial of an educational program to prevent low back injuries. [See comments.] *New England Journal of Medicine* 337 (5; July 31, 1997): 322–28.

Additional study showing back care education had no effect on people who had already developed pain:

Berwick, D. M.; Budman, S.; Feldstein, M. No clinical effect of back schools in an HMO: A randomized prospective trial. *Spine* 14 (3; Mar. 1989): 338–44.

Review of medical literature on back school programs showing that they have no apparent benefit:

Linton, S. J.; Kamwendo, K. Low back schools: A critical review. *Physical Therapy* 67 (9; Sept. 1987): 1375–83.

CHAPTER 8

Examples of how phobias are cured with exposure and response prevention—snake phobia example (sidebar):

Hepner, A.; Cauthen, N. R.; Effect of subject control and graduated exposure on snake phobias. *Journal of Consulting and Clinical Psychology* 43 (3; June 1975): 297–304.

Russell, R. K.; Mathews, C. O. Cue-controlled relaxation in vivo desensitization of a snake phobia. *Journal of Behavioral Therapy and Experimental Psychiatry* 6 (1; Apr. 1975): 49–51.

Gate-control theory of pain:

Melzak, R.; Wall, P. D. Pain mechanisms: A new theory. *Science* 50 (1965): 971–79.

Fear of pain involves different brain regions than the pain itself (sidebar):

Fear of pain may be worse than pain itself. *New York Times*, June 22, 1999.

CHAPTER 9

Research showing that even short bouts of back pain make people feel frustrated:

Philips, H. C.; Grant, L. Acute back pain: A psychological analysis. *Behaviour Research and Therapy* 29 (5; 1991): 429–34.

Research showing suppressing anger has serious health consequences:

See sources under chapter 10, first four citations.

Research showing that people suffering from depression and chronic pain think negatively, often *catastrophizing:*

Estlander, A.; Haerkaepaeae, K. Relationships between coping strategies, disability and pain levels in patients with chronic low back pain. *Scandinavian Journal of Behavioural Therapy* 18 (2; 1989): 59–69.

Sullivan, M. J. L.; Stanish, W.; Waite, H.; Sullivan, M.; Tripp, D. Catas–trophizing, pain, and disability in patients with soft-tissue injuries. *Pain* 77 (3; Sept. 1998): 253–60.

Research showing that people with chronic pain make other cognitive errors, such as *overgeneralizing,* which lead to a negative outlook:

Lefebvre, M. F. Cognitive distortion and cognitive errors in depressed psychiatric and low back pain patients. *Journal of Consulting and Clinical Psychology* 49 (4; Aug. 1981): 517–25.

Smith, T. W.; Follick, M. J.; Ahern, D. K.; Adams A. Cognitive distortion and disability in chronic low back pain. *Cognitive Therapy and Research* 10 (2; Apr. 1986): 201–10.

CHAPTER 10

People who don't notice their negative emotions have increased heart rates, suffer from weakened immune system reactions, feel physically ill, and visit the doctor more than those who acknowledge these feelings:

Schwartz, G. E. Psychobiology of repression and health: A systems approach. In Singer, J. L. (ed.). *Repression and dissociation: Defense mechanisms and personality styles: Current theory and research.* Chicago: University of Chicago Press, 1990: 405–34.

Study showing that suppressing anger in particular contributes to chronic, disabling headaches:

Hatch J. P.; Schoeinfeld L. S.; Boutros N. N.; Seleshi E.; et al. Anger and hostility in tension-type headache. *Headache* 31 (5; May 1991): 302–4.

Study showing that back pain sufferers who suppress anger have the greatest increases in back muscle tension when put in anger-provoking situations:

Burns, J. W. Anger management style and hostility: Predicting symptom-specific physiological reactivity among chronic low back pain patients. *Journal of Behavioral Medicine* 20 (6; Dec. 1997): 505–22.

Research showing that anxiety problems are most common in people who don't acknowledge or express negative emotions:

Shear, M. K.; Weiner, K. Psychotherapy for panic disorder. *Journal of Clinical Psychiatry* 58 (Supp. 2; 1997): 38–45.

Research indicating which life events are generally the most stressful:

Holmes, T. H.; Rahe, R. H. The social readjustment rating scale. *Journal of Psychosomatic Research* 11 (2; 1967): 213–18.

Panic attacks don't actually come on "out of the blue" but are preceded by events that cause sadness, anger, or fear:

Milrod, B.; Busch, F. N.; Hollander, E.; Aronson, A.; et al. A 23-year-old woman with panic disorder treated with psychodynamic psychotherapy. *American Journal of Psychiatry* 153 (5; May 1996): 698–703.

Shear, M. K.; Weiner, K. Psychotherapy for panic disorder. *Journal of Clinical Psychiatry* 58 (Supp. 2; 1997): 38–45.

Examples of studies suggesting that assertiveness reduces stress responses:

Petrie, K.; Rotheram, M. J. Insulators against stress: Self-esteem and assertiveness. *Psychological Reports* 50 (3, Pt. 1; June 1982): 963–66.

Tomaka, J.; Palacios, R.; Schneider, K. T.; Colotla, M.; Concha, J. B.; Herrald, M. Assertiveness predicts threat and challenge reactions to potential stress among women. *Journal of Personality and Social Psychology* 76 (6; June 1999): 1008–21.

Study indicating that assertiveness augments the benefits of social support for psychological adjustment:

Elliott, T. R.; Gramling, S. E. Personal assertiveness and the effects of social support among college students. *Journal of Counseling Psychology* 37 (4; Oct. 1990): 427–36.

Study showing that more assertive people have fewer health problems:

Williams, J. M.; Stout, J. K. The effect of high and low assertiveness on locus of control and health problems. *Journal of Psychology* 119 (2; Mar. 1985): 169–73.

Study showing that training in assertiveness helps to reduce stress:

Lee, S.; Crockett, M. S. Effect of assertiveness training on levels of stress and assertiveness experienced by nurses in Taiwan, Republic of China. *Issues in Mental Health Nursing* 15 (4; July–Aug. 1994): 419–32.

Venting anger is fraught with difficulties (sidebar):

Letting out aggression is called bad advice. *New York Times*, Mar. 9, 1999.

Personal health. *New York Times*, Nov. 20, 1996.

Journal writing reduced visits to health services and enhanced immune system functioning:

Pennebaker, J. W.; Keicolt-Glaser, J. K.; Glaser, R. Disclosure of traumas and immune function: Health implications for psychotherapy. *Journal of Consulting and Clinical Psychology* 56 (2; Apr. 1988): 239–45.

Journal writing produced lasting improvements in asthma and arthritis symptoms:

Smyth, J. M.; Stone, A. A.; Hurewitz, A.; Kaell, A. Effects of writing about stressful experiences on symptom reduction in patients with asthma or rheumatoid arthritis: A randomized trial. *JAMA* 281 (14; Apr. 1999): 1304–9.

Examples of other studies showing positive effects of journal writing on health measures:

Francis, M. E.; Pennebaker, J. W. Putting stress into words: The impact of writing on physiological, absentee, and self-reported emotional well-being measures. *American Journal of Health Promotion* 64 (4; Mar.–Apr. 1992): 280–87.

Petrie, K. J.; Booth, R. J.; Pennebaker, J. W. The immunological effects of thought suppression. *Journal of Personality and Social Psychology* 75 (5; Nov. 1998): 1264–72.

Study showing that people who become disabled by chronic back pain tend to have a family history of the same problem:

Pollard, C. A. Family history and severity of disability associated with chronic low back pain. *Psychological Reports* 57 (3, Pt. 1; Dec. 1985): 813–14.

Examples of studies showing that spouses of people with chronic back pain themselves become depressed and experience marital dissatisfaction:

Ahern, D. K.; Follick, M. J. Distress in spouses of chronic pain patients. *International Journal of Family Therapy* 7 (4; Winter 1985): 247–57.

Schwartz, L.; Slater, M. A.; Birchler, G. R.; Atkinson, J. H. Depression in spouses of chronic pain patients: The role of patient pain and anger, and marital satisfaction. *Pain* 44 (1; Jan. 1991): 61–67.

Study showing that sexual difficulties following back pain cause marital stress:

Ferroni, P. A.; Coates, R. Blue-collar workers: Back injury and its effect on family life. *Australian Journal of Sex, Marriage and Family* 10 (1; Feb. 1989): 5–11.

Study indicating that marriages generally survived despite the far-reaching effects of chronic back pain:

Humphrey, M.; Jones, N. Chronic pain and marital stability. *Stress Medicine* 3 (4; Oct.–Dec. 1987): 261–62.

Stressful interactions with a spouse cause back pain patients to give up on physical activity:

Schwartz, L.; Slater, M. A.; Birchler, G. R. Interpersonal stress and pain behaviors in patients with chronic pain. *Journal of Consulting and Clinical Psychology* 62 (4; Aug. 1994): 861–64.

Positive social interaction allowed chronic back pain patients to persist with a lifting task:

Fisher, K.; Johnston, M. Emotional distress as a mediator of the relationship between pain and disability: An experimental study. *British Journal of Health Psychology* 1 (Pt. 3; Sept. 1996): 207–18.

CHAPTER 11

People with back pain often suffer from other muscle or joint pain and have high rates of health care use:

Rekola, K. E.; Keinaenen-Kiukaanniemi, S.; Takal, J. Use of health services by patients seeking care for low back pain symptoms: A population-based prospective study of consultations with primary care physicians. *Journal of Musculoskeletal Pain* 1 (2; 1993): 55–64.

Nonrestorative sleep is common in a variety of muscle pain disorders:

Davidson, P. *Chronic muscle pain syndrome.* New York: Berkley Publishing Group, 1994.

A good review of insomnia:

Kupfer, D. J.; Reynolds, C. F.; III. Management of insomnia. *New England Journal of Medicine* 336 (5; Jan. 30, 1997): 341–46.

Study showing that 60 percent of women with chronic back pain reported having been sexually abused as children:

Pecukonis, E. V. Childhood sex abuse in women with chronic intractable back pain. *Social Work in Health Care* 23 (3; 1996): 1–16.

Holocaust survivors report more chronic pain than other subjects:

Yaari, A.; Eisenberg, E.; Adler, R.; Birkhan, J. Chronic pain in Holocaust survivors. *Journal of Pain and Symptom Management* 17 (3; Mar. 1999): 181–87.

Vietnam combat veterans with post-traumatic stress disorder had high levels of chronic back pain:

Beckham, J. C.; Crawford, A. L.; Feldman, M. E.; Kirby, A. C.; Hertzberg, M. A.; et al. Chronic post-traumatic stress disorder and chronic pain in Vietnam combat veterans. *Journal of Psychosomatic Research* 43 (3; Oct. 1997): 379–89.

Examples of further studies showing higher reports of childhood abuse in adults suffering from chronic back pain:

Blair, J. A.; Blair, R. S.; Rueckert, P. Pre-injury emotional trauma and chronic back pain: An unexpected finding. *Spine* 19 (10; May 15, 1994): 1144–46.

Linton, S. J. A population-based study of the relationship between sexual abuse and back pain: Establishing a link. *Pain* 73 (1; Oct. 1997): 47–53.

Schofferman, J.; Anderson, D.; Hines, R.; Smith, G.; Keane, G. Childhood psychological trauma and chronic refractory low-back pain. *Clinical Journal of Pain* 4 (Dec. 1993): 260–65.

People with a number of anxiety or stress-related problems are more likely than other people to have suffered through difficult times as a child:

Shear, M. K.; Weiner, K. Psychotherapy for panic disorder. *Journal of Clinical Psychiatry* 58 (Supp. 2; 1997): 38–45.

Examples of research studies showing that disability payments interfere with recovery from chronic back pain:

Gatchel R. J.; Polatin, P. B.; Mayer, T. G. The dominant role of psychosocial risk factors in the development of chronic low back pain disability. *Spine* 20 (24; Dec. 15, 1995): 2702–9.

Gentry, W. D.; Shows, W. D.; Thomas, M. Chronic low back pain: A psychological profile. *Psychosomatics* 15 (4; 1974): 174–77.

Rainville, J.; Sobel, J. B.; Hartigan, C.; Wright, A. The effect of compensation involvement on the reporting of pain and disability by patients referred for rehabilitation of chronic low back pain. *Spine* 22 (17; Sept. 1, 1997): 2016–24.

Rohling, M. L.; Binder, L. M.; Langhinrichsen-Rohling, J. Money matters: A meta-analytic review of the association between financial compensation and the experience and treatment of chronic pain. *Health Psychology* 14 (6; Nov. 1995): 537–47.

CHAPTER 12

Research involving the health benefits of the relaxation response:

Benson, H.; Klipper, M. Z. The relaxation response. New York: Avon Books, 2000.

Research demonstrating that mindfulness meditation is helpful for chronic pain:

Kabat-Zinn J.; Lipworth L.; Burney, R. The clinical use of mindfulness meditation for the self-regulation of chronic pain. *Journal of Behavioral Medicine* (2; June 8, 1985): 163–190.

Randolph P. D.; Caldera Y. M.; Tacon A. M.; Greak B. L. The long-term combined effects of medical treatment and a mindfulness-based behavioral program for the multidisciplinary management of chronic pain in West Texas. *Pain Digest* 9 (1999): 103–12.

Research demonstrating that mindfulness meditation is helpful for other stress-related problems:

Kabat-Zinn, J.; Wheeler, E.; Light, T.; Skillings, A.; Scharf, M. J.; Cropley, T. G.; Hosmer, D.; Bernhard, J. D. Influence of a mindfulness meditation-based stress reduction intervention on rates of skin-clearing in patients with moderate to severe psoriasis undergoing phototherapy (UVB) and photochemotherapy (PUVA). *Psychosomatic Medicine* 60 (5; Sept.–Oct. 1998): 625–32.

Miller, J. J.; Fletcher, K.; Kabat-Zinn, J. Three-year follow-up and clinical implications of a mindfulness meditation-based stress reduction intervention in the treatment of anxiety disorders. *General Hospital Psychiatry* 17 (3; May 1995): 192–200.

Dealing with pain through distraction may actually make the pain worse later:

Cioffi, D.; Holloway, J. Delayed costs of suppressed pain. *Journal of Personality and Social Psychology* 64 (2; Feb. 1993): 274–82.

"If you have a mind, it is going to wander." Quote from Jon Kabat-Zinn found in:

Domar, A. D.; Dreher, H. *Healing mind, healthy woman: Using the mind-body connection to manage stress and take control of your life.* New York: Doubleday, 1997: 63.

People who feel supported by their religion have better odds of recovering from many illnesses (sidebar):

Paths to a higher plane and longer life. *New York Times,* Aug. 17, 1999.

Religious practices positively influence health:

Larson, D. B. *The faith factor: An annotated bibliography of systematic reviews and clinical research on spiritual subjects.* Vol. II. John Templeton Foundation, 1993.

Levin, J. S. Religion and health: Is there an association, is it valid, and is it causal? *Social Science and Medicine* 38 (11; June 1994): 1475–82.

HMOs are using mindfulness techniques to treat stress-related disorders (sidebar):

Health maintenance organizations turn to spiritual healing. *New York Times,* Dec. 27, 1995.

CHAPTER 13

Research supporting safety and efficacy of aggressive exercise programs:

See citations under chapter 7, Rainville; Mitchell; and chapter 4, Mayer.

Overviews of exercise prescription:

Guidelines for exercise testing and prescription/American College of Sports Medicine, 6th ed. Philadelphia: Lea and Feibiger, 2000.

SAM-CD The Scientific American Medicine CD-ROM. New York: *Scientific American*, 1999: chapter 4, "Diet and Exercise."

APPENDIX 1

Reviews of back pain diagnosis and treatment, including demographics, findings, prognosis:

Bigos, S.; Bowyer, O.; Braen, G.; et al. Acute low back problems in adults. Clinical Practice Guideline No. 14. AHCPR Publication No. 95–0642. Rockville, MD: Agency for Health Care Policy and Research, Public Health Service, U.S. Department of Health and Human Services. December 1994.

Frymoyer, J. W. Back pain and sciatica. *New England Journal of Medicine* 318 (5; Feb. 4, 1988): 291–300.

Waddell, G. 1987 Volvo award in clinical sciences. A new clinical model for the treatment of low-back pain. *Spine* 12 (7; Sept. 1987): 632–44.

APPENDIX 2

Comment on that back pain treatment follows "fads":

Deyo, R. A. Fads in the treatment of low back pain [editorial; comment]. *New England Journal of Medicine* 325 (14; Oct. 3, 1991): 1039–40.

Reviews of back pain treatments:

See citations under appendix 1.

INDEX